Amazing Essential Oils
MAKE & TAKES

Amazing Essential Oils
MAKE & TAKES

144 DIY IDEAS FOR HOSTING
THE PERFECT CLASS

DONNA RASKIN

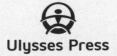

Ulysses Press

Published in the United States by:
Ulysses Press
P.O. Box 3440
Berkeley, CA 94703
www.ulyssespress.com

ISBN: 978-1-61243-837-5
Library of Congress Catalog Number 2018944066

Printed in Canada by Marquis Book Printing
10 9 8 7 6 5 4 3 2 1

Acquisitions editor: Casie Vogel
Managing editor: Claire Chun
Editor: Shayna Keyles
Proofreader: Barbara Schultz
Cover design: Raquel Castro
Artwork: cover © 279photo Studio/shutterstock.com; season icons
    © lettett/shutterstock.com
Production: Jake Flaherty, Claire Sielaff

Distributed by Publishers Group West

Contents

MEDICINE CABINET......................................60

Introduction

When people walk into my home, they often stop and say, "It smells good in here." They take a deep breath and, after they exhale, they smile. Immediately, the aroma calms them, and we sit to have tea and talk.

The essential oils I have in diffusers, simple clay bowls, and candles around my home help to create a mood, just as much as my furniture, baking, and tea or coffee do when a friend visits. Like you, I want to be hospitable. I want people to come into my home and feel comfortable immediately, and one of the easiest and least expensive ways to achieve this is with essential oils.

In the case of essential oils, the word "essential" means "essence." In other words, the oils are the very "essence" of rose or lavender or grapefruit. An essential oil is not an imitation or synthetic. More importantly, though, the essence of an essential oil is a key to its power. Scent is directly related to our "sense" of memory and mood. Although it's true that the human sense of smell is not as strong as that of a dog, it is also true that we respond to scent in a more subtle, and yet still powerful, manner.

For example, our sense of smell is 10,000 times more powerful than our sense of taste. In fact, much of what we consider taste is truly our sense of smell. Think about when you have the flu and make a pot of homemade chicken soup. Most of us first inhale the scent of the soup before we eat. Both the steam and the aroma of the chicken, carrots, and onions are immediately soothing and healing.

Interestingly, scientists have long believed that much of our response to aroma is based on association rather than cause and effect. For example, that chicken soup I just described—it is not so much that the smell of onions immediately works to cure the flu, but that because we associate the scent of chicken soup with healing, our minds begin to focus on the act of healing once we have the chicken soup in front of us.

However, traditional medicine experts, and now many holistic medical specialists, understand that the essential oils themselves, and not just their scent, have curative powers. For example, tea tree oil, which comes from the *Melaleuca alternifolia* plant, which is native to Australia, has long been an effective antifungal and antivirus medication. In other words, while it is a fragrant essential oil, it is not just its scent that improves our health. Tea tree oil kills bacteria on human skin and kills mold in the atmosphere, among other uses, so its scent is secondary to its other healing properties.

Most people who are new to essential oils think their value comes predominantly from their scents and the way we feel when we smell the oil, but that's not entirely true. Many essential oils have other medicinal qualities and can be applied to the skin or taken internally. However, since I am not a doctor and because I can't guarantee the quality of the oils you purchase, I don't feel comfortable recommending you take any oils internally or use uncommon ones on your skin to be absorbed.

Making Essential Oils Gifts and Projects

Let's face it, in the face of the pharmaceutical and medical industries, essential oils are a small informal business. Essential oil experts don't visit dermatologists to give samples and suggest that they offer their customers tea tree oil rather than a new, expensive-to-develop, chemical acne medicine. They don't tell a child psychologist that there is scientific backing to suggest that a teenager light a home-made aromatherapy candle with orange and peppermint to help her focus while she studies.

The fact is, essential oils and aromatherapy may not be high-tech or pharmaceutical, but they work. (See page 153 for answers to frequently asked questions about essential oils.) Plus, they are inexpensive and we can learn about them through experience, both hands-on and anecdotal. For example, I had a massage therapist who used the most incredible lavender and eucalyptus oil and I still use that mixture to help me relax. I have friends who use Etsy to buy homemade candles made with ylang-ylang and bergamot to create an atmosphere of romance. More than anything, though, essential oils are easy to experiment with and learn from on your own.

All around you, people are using essential oils. Many of these people want to learn more recipes and craft ideas so they can give essential oil gifts or sell essential oils and their products. Candles, diffuser mixtures, medicine cabinet recipes, beauty products, and holiday presents—these are just some of the fun creations you and your friends, and eventually your customers, can make with essential oils.

Essential Oil Party How-Tos

Hosting an essential oil party is a great way to introduce your friends and family to the benefits of essential oils. Like any party, your event will be more successful if you take certain steps.

First, try to focus not on selling, but on sharing information, just the way a teacher does. You have a passion for essential oils, and, just like a school teacher, you want your guests, or students, to learn more about your passion so that they will share it, as well.

I'm a teacher, and the first thing I always do is ask questions. This immediately engages your guest. You might start with, "Have any you ever walked into a room and immediately noticed the scent? Do you remember what it was?" If one of your guests answers, try to pull out the scent that they mention. If it was flowers, take out your orange blossom oil, while if it was the smell of cookies in the kitchen, let them sniff your vanilla essential oil. Make sure it is passed around so everyone gets to smell.

As they smell the oils, ask them what they notice about how it feels to inhale the scent. People aren't good with descriptive words (teachers know this; if you ask anyone if they liked a book or movie, they will usually say, "It was good"), so be ready to supply them with some adjectives to make them aware of their improved mood. *Do you feel a little calmer? Do you feel happier? Do you remember a relaxing day with your family?*

Then, begin to explain why essential oils are good for us, but be sure not to oversell them. Essential oils aren't miracle cures, but they are helpful for both our mood and our health. You might tell your guests that some essential oils, such as tea tree and myrrh, can fight infections. Some fight inflammation and are good for our skin, such as rose and cedarwood, while others lift our mood, such as lavender and geranium. You might make little cards for each oil so that your customers can easily see the oils' benefits.

Also, remember that human beings naturally respond to stories. So instead of simply saying, for example, "Rose essential oil is good for your skin," it is far more effective to say, "My friend Kristi had terrible rosacea and she made a lotion with rose and geranium oil. She used it every day and the rosacea cleared up in two weeks."

If you feel like you don't have enough stories to tell, I have introduced almost every one of these recipes with a story of my own, so feel free to say, "My friend Donna...." The point of this book is for you to use the recipes both on your own and when you host a Make-and-Take party. My stories may help you remember (or create!) stories of your own.

How to Use This Book

The projects in this book are organized by category, difficulty, and season. Each chapter is a different type of project, like Home or Family. Within each chapter, projects are labeled by season and difficulty. Each project is labeled by season because, like the plants and flowers from which they derive, I think of oils as seasonal. For example, there are a lot of woodsy scents in winter and floral aromas in spring. You'll see an icon on the side of each page letting you know the season of each project:

 is a spring project

 is a summer project

 is a fall project

 is a winter project

Also, in each chapter, recipes are organized from Easy to Hard. All of the Easy and Medium recipes work as make-and-take projects, while the Hard projects are perfect recipes to share with your customers or make as gifts.

When you choose a recipe, decide if you are making enough for everyone before they get to the party, or if people will be making the recipes themselves while they're all together. Either way, you're going to have to figure out two things: First, how to multiply the recipe to get the number of make-and-takes you will need, and second, how you are going to send the recipes home. I didn't include packaging instructions for each recipe; for example, some of the bath recipes simply suggest adding blends into running water. If you want to turn a bath recipe into a make-and-take or a gift, you might need to buy glass bottles or small Mason jars and ribbon to make them extra cute.

Multiplying ingredients for recipes is not an exact science. You may use a bigger glass bottle than I would use, or you might like a recipe where one essential oil is stronger than another. Personalizing these recipes is fun. Play with them! I am partial to grapefruit, but maybe you are partial to orange. You can usually substitute a citrus for a citrus or a floral for a floral.

Finally, let's say that you're going on a spa weekend with your friends. You can certainly take a shaving cream recipe that I created for men and turn it into a more traditional feminine scent by changing the cedarwood to ylang-ylang, for example. Remember, though, that the number of drops needed for one scent will not exactly match the number of drops needed for another. You may need to experiment to find the right balance.

Similarly, different essential oils have different health benefits, but that doesn't mean you can't substitute one essential oil for another. So while lemon energizes and neroli is soothing, that doesn't mean you shouldn't see what happens when you switch them around in a body lotion or diffuser.

Materials You'll Need

- Air-drying clay
- Baking sheets
- Beeswax
- Bowls
- Cheesecloth
- Chopsticks

- Cookie cutters or craft knives
- Cotton wicks
- Double boiler reserved for crafts
- Epsom salts
- Fabric
- Funnels
- Glass dropper bottles
- Liquid measuring cups
- Mason jars
- Needle and thread
- Paper
- Pencils
- Potato masher
- Pots reserved for crafts
- Pre-cut cloth facial masks
- Rags
- Ramekins
- Ribbon or cord
- Roller bottles
- Rolling pin
- Sandpaper
- Silicone molds (e.g., Easter egg mold)
- Spray bottles
- Thread
- Towels

- Various-sized cosmetic tubes
- Washcloths
- Whisks
- Wooden spoon reserved for crafts

Around the House

Vinegar and Grapefruit Window Cleaner

For many years, I lived in a three-story house that faced the Atlantic Ocean. The windows were huge and the views were perfect, so, of course, my windows had to be pristine. The secret was this window cleaner, which not only kept the glass transparent, but also beautifully scented the house. This is a great make-and-take hostess gift, as you can put it in smaller bottles and give it a creative name.

LEVEL: Easy

MAKES: 1 (24-ounce) spray bottle

Ingredients

⅔ cup white vinegar

⅓ cup rubbing alcohol

1 cup filtered water

10 drops grapefruit essential oil

1. Put a funnel in the top of a clean spray bottle and pour the ingredients into a spray bottle.

2. Gently shake the bottle and spray on the window, using newspaper or a lint-free cloth to wipe away. Shake the bottle before each use.

TIP: If grapefruit is not a scent you enjoy, any citrus essential oil is perfect as a window cleaner.

Lavender Kitchen Degreaser

If you're tired of the typical citrus oil kitchen scent, you might want to try this recipe with lavender, which is more relaxing than orange or lemon.

LEVEL: Easy

MAKES: 1 (24-ounce) glass bottle

Ingredients

2 cups warm water

1 tablespoon baking soda

20 drops lavender
essential oil

¼ cup white vinegar

¼ cup natural liquid soap

1. Mix 2 cups of warm water, 1 tablespoon of baking soda, and 20 drops lavender essential oil.

2. Add white vinegar and natural soap.

3. Funnel the mixture into a spray bottle.

4. Spray the mixture on grease and let sit for about 30 seconds. Then, wipe with a damp towel.

Tea Tree and Lemon Floor Cleaner

One day while I was using my Swiffer, I thought about spraying some essential oils onto the Swiffer sheets to improve their use. What could be better than scenting the house while I cleaned?

LEVEL: Medium

MAKES: 1 (8-ounce) spray bottle

Ingredients

1 cup distilled water

2 tablespoons white distilled vinegar

2 tablespoons rubbing alcohol

10 drops tea tree oil

10 drops lemon oil

1. Mix the water, vinegar, and alcohol in a measuring cup. Add the essential oils.

2. Funnel the mixture into a spray bottle.

3. When using your Swiffer (dry or wet), spray the mixture onto the cloth and use as you normally would.

Living Room Orange Blossom Hydrosol

Orange blossom is the distillation of a flower sometimes called sour orange, so its scent is not quite like the orange we eat. It's a little greener and less sharp, and it has more depth. The scent is calming. The same plant also makes neroli and petitgrain. For a make-and-take party, package in 4-ounce spray bottles (you can often find them in blue, which is extra pretty) and write the project title on a pretty label.

LEVEL: Easy

MAKES: 1 (4-ounce) glass spray bottle

Ingredients

filtered water

10 drops orange blossom essential oil

1. Fill a spray bottle with filtered water. Add the orange blossom oil. Shake gently and thoroughly.

2. Spray up and in the middle of the room to allow the scent to diffuse throughout the room.

TIP: If you're making this as a project for your make-and-take party, put guests' names and some decorations on the bottles before they arrive.

Tea Tree and Lavender After Gardening Facial Wipe

When I've been working outside, I am often too tired to wash my face well afterward, but I always want to cool off (and clean off!), too. My solution? I use a washcloth, which is more earth-friendly than a disposable wipe. I start a bottle before I head outside and then, when I come in, I have an easy way to clean up. For a gift, you could package a jar containing the ingredients with two decorative washcloths.

LEVEL: Hard

MAKES: 2 washcloths

Ingredients

¼ cup water

2 tablespoons witch hazel

10 drops tea tree essential oil

10 drops lavender essential oil

2 washcloths

1. Before you go outside to work, mix the water, witch hazel, and essential oils in a liquid measuring cup. Put the washcloths in a jar with a lid and pour the liquid over the washcloths.

2. Put a lid on the jar and very gently shake so that the washcloths soak in the liquid. You can also use a spoon or fork to move the washcloths in the jar. Cover the jar and put it in the refrigerator before you go outside.

3. When you come back inside, get the jar. Wash your hands, get out a washcloth, and squeeze it gently over the sink so it drips less. Use it on your face, chest, neck, and arms (or anywhere else you were sweating).

Rose Friendship Candle

This is wonderful giveaway for guests at a make-and-take party. You can make a batch and pour them into small Mason jars so you don't have to use that much of your essential oils. The amount of essential oil you use depends on the strength of the oil's scent, whether the oils are being mixed together, and the amount of wax you use. I like to mix in the essential oil until I can smell it, and then add a few more drops.

LEVEL: Hard

MAKES: 6 (8-ounce) candles

Ingredients

6 (8-ounce) Mason jars

double boiler

3 pounds organic beeswax

25 drops rose essential oil

15 drops jasmine essential oil

15 drops sweet orange essential oil

natural food coloring (optional)

6 cotton wicks

6 pencils

1. Clean the Mason jars and dry them thoroughly.

2. Put water in the bottom of a double boiler, place the boiler on the stove, and turn on the heat until the water reaches a simmer.

3. Place beeswax in the top part of the boiler until it melts, about 5 minutes over low heat. Once it has melted, remove it from the heat and stir in the essential oils. Add food color, if using, one drop at a time, until desired color is achieved.

4. Cut the wicks to be twice the size of your clean Mason jars. Tape one end of each wick the middle of a pencil or stick, wrap the wick around the pencil a few times, and then let it hang over and into the jar.

5. Slowly pour the wax into the Mason jars so the wax covers the wick. Leave the wick in place and put the candle in a cool location. Cover lightly with a towel and let it harden for a day.

6. When the wax has hardened, cut the wick to the right length.

Vegetable Plant Insect Repellent Spray

Having a "Make-and-Take Garden Party" is a great summertime idea, and this recipe is an inexpensive one you can give your guests as their take home gift. You can pair it with a tomato plant or packet of seeds. You can spray this on tomatoes, lettuces, cabbages, and other produce, making sure you wash vegetables thoroughly before you eat them or cook them.

LEVEL: Easy

MAKES: 1 (8-ounce) spray bottle

Ingredients

5 drops rosemary oil

5 drops peppermint oil

5 drops thyme oil

5 drops clove oil

1 cup water

Put the oils and the water in a spray bottle and shake, then spray. Shake before each use to make sure the oils aren't settling in the water.

TIP: One of the most potent natural insecticides is neem oil, which kills many parasites by dissolving their waxy skin. Neem oil also kills larvae and eggs, so it stops the continued infestation. There's just one problem. Neem oil does not smell good. So, while it is fine to use in the garden, you might not want to use it on plants in your house. The spray above is a great alternative.

Summer Potpourri Sachet

Sometimes it's difficult for me to go to work on summer days. I'd rather be down the shore! One thing that helps is surrendering to the heat and humidity of New Jersey and doing all I can to stay cool, and that includes lightly perfuming my lingerie by keeping these sachets in my drawers (get it?). This is a great sewing project for kids!

LEVEL: Hard

MAKES: 1 sachet

Ingredients

4 x 8-inch piece of muslin

needle and thread

¼ cup dried roses

½ cup flaxseeds

20 drops rose essential oil

1. Fold the muslin in half, so the outside faces inward.

2. Sew the two side ends together tightly and sew most of the top, leaving an inch or so open to put in the potpourri.

3. Mix the roses, flaxseeds, and essential oil together in a small bowl, and add the mixture into the sachet using a spoon.

4. Tightly sew the rest of the sachet. Place in your clothes drawers.

Grapefruit and Geranium Kitchen Degreaser

I'll be honest, I am neither Betty Crocker nor Mr. Clean, so things like the knobs on my stove can become...not ideal. This degreaser is perfect for those types of spaces. I would bring this as a housewarming gift. You could also use this recipe for guests at a housewarming make-and-take party and have your guests use their favorite essential oil combinations to personalize their recipes.

LEVEL: Easy

MAKES: 1 (16-ounce) bottle

Ingredients

1 cup white vinegar

12 drops grapefruit essential oil

12 drops geranium essential oil

1 cup baking soda

1. Mix the white vinegar and essential oils in a spray bottle.

2. To use, put the baking soda in a ramekin or small bowl. Spray the essential oil solution onto the greasy surface and let sit for a few seconds. Then, dip a small part of a rag into the baking soda. Scrub the area you sprayed.

3. Wet with water to get the baking soda off, and then dry.

Vinegar and Orange Window Cleaner

I know I'm the only person who still reads newspapers, but they really are the best way to clean glass, especially if you use this cleaner with the papers.

LEVEL: Easy

MAKES: 1 (16-ounce) spray bottle

Ingredients

2 cups filtered water

¼ cup rubbing alcohol

¼ cup distilled white vinegar

½ teaspoon orange essential oil

Add all ingredients to a spray bottle and shake to mix. To use, spray on a glass surface and wipe with a page of newspaper.

Grapefruit and Geranium Room Freshener

Essential oil room fresheners are not like the aerosol sprays that hurt the environment, which is to say, you can't just spray them around the room and have them "dissipate." Essential oil room fresheners also don't use power like the plug-in variety. These are two of the reasons I like to use all-natural room fresheners like this one. I spray it on stain-resistant fabrics, such as my rug. In the summer, I spray it toward my fans or air conditioner. Essential oils don't stain, but you don't want them to land in a puddle in your furniture or good fabrics.

LEVEL: Easy

MAKES: 1 (4-ounce) spray bottle

Ingredients

½ cup alcohol

20 drops lemon essential oil

20 drops basil essential oil

Pour alcohol and essential oils in a spray bottle. Close lid and shake gently to combine. To use, spray on surfaces that can handle alcohol, which will evaporate.

Grapefruit and Geranium Dishwasher Powder

We forget that just a few generations ago people didn't have an enormous grocery store aisle from which to choose soap for their dishwasher. There was just powder and it didn't come in a variety of scents. You can use this baking "soap," which is actually called "washing soda," to create an environmentally friendly dishwashing product that smells the way you want and isn't expensive. You can find washing soda online (and you'll recognize the brand names).

LEVEL: Medium

MAKES: 1 large Mason jar (about 12 washes)

Ingredients

1 cup washing soda

½ cup salt

½ cup citric acid

25 drops lemon essential oil

1. Mix all ingredients very well in a Mason jar with a lid.

2. When you want to use, scoop out two tablespoons powder and put in dishwasher. Run the dishwasher. You might have to experiment with how much you need based on your dishes and whether your water is hard or soft.

Fruit and Vegetable Wash

I eat a lot of fruits and vegetables, and although I try to buy locally from nearby organic farms, I shop in a supermarket every Sunday, so I end up purchasing plenty of produce that has been sprayed from seed to picking. I keep this wash on my kitchen counter and use it with all of my produce. Rather than soaking, I spray some of this wash on my produce and rinse with tap water. Be sure to dry with a towel or air dry all of your produce before storing.

LEVEL: Easy

MAKES: 1 (12-ounce) bottle

Ingredients

    1 cup distilled water

    ⅓ cup white vinegar

    15 drops lemon essential oil

Add all the ingredients to a large spray bottle. Shake well.

TIP: If you use this wash with berries, line a baking sheet with paper towel, spread the berries on the sheet, and cover with clean dishcloth. Then, put in the refrigerator for an hour. When they are dry, you can put them in a bowl or plastic storage dish.

Grapefruit and Geranium Scrubbing Cleaner

This cleanser scrubs well but isn't rough, so you can use it in tubs or even stainless steel sinks. The essential oils you add will even help with the disinfecting!

LEVEL: Medium

MAKES: 1 large Mason jar (2 cups)

Ingredients

1 cup baking soda

¼ cup Castile soap

2 tablespoons hydrogen peroxide

20 drops tea tree essential oil

10 drops lemon essential oil

1. Combine the baking soda, soap, and peroxide, but don't overmix, as you don't want the baking soda to dissolve.

2. Add the essential oils and mix gently.

3. Put the scrub in a large Mason jar, but do not fully seal. Be sure to leave room for the scrub to grow (the baking soda feeds on the hydrogen).

4. To use, put about a tablespoon of the scrub on a damp sponge, dampen the surface to be cleaned, and scrub gently. Wipe away any excess.

Grapefruit and Geranium Multipurpose Spray

You might want to play with this recipe a bit to see how soapy you like your cleanser. I find I need more Castile soap than others do because my kitchen counters and oven/stove seem to be greasy. But, you can make this without the soap if you want. It will certainly wipe away anything on glass or a countertop.

LEVEL: Easy

MAKES: 1 (16-ounce) spray bottle

Ingredients

¼ cup white vinegar

1¾ cups water

2 tablespoons Castile soap

15 drops grapefruit essential oil

15 drops geranium essential oil

Add all ingredients to a large spray bottle. Shake gently, then spray on counter or glass and wipe away.

TIP: I wouldn't use this on wood, but it's OK to use on plastics, linoleum, and glass.

Grapefruit and Geranium Shower Spray

My mother keeps a squeegee and glass cleaner in her shower. It's like taking a shower in a car wash. I simply use homemade shower spray every few days. No squeegee needed. If you want to give cleaning products as gifts, or if you want to have your clients make them as gifts, I suggest you also talk to them about labeling and include that activity as part of your get-together. For example, cleaning and beauty product ingredients need to be clearly labeled, and it's nice to have a common design element on all the products. Even homemade products benefit from easy-to-read print and an icon or picture that represents the seller's point of view.

LEVEL: Easy

MAKES: 1 (16-ounce) spray bottle

Ingredients

2 cups water

1 ½ cups white vinegar

½ cup rubbing alcohol

1 tablespoon Castile soap

20 drops grapefruit essential oil

20 drops geranium essential oil

10 drops tea tree essential oil

1. Mix all the ingredients in a bowl, then funnel the mixture into a large spray bottle.

2. To use, spray on the shower glass or wall, let sit for a few seconds, then wipe away.

Citrus and Cedarwood Carpet Freshener

One of the few things I do right in terms of housecleaning is vacuuming (the other is laundry, but no one turns to me for dishes or dusting), and this carpet freshener is one of my secrets. It vacuums up easily and it leaves the house smelling fantastic!

LEVEL: Medium
MAKES: 1 use

Ingredients

2 cups baking soda

10 drops sweet orange oil

10 drops cedarwood oil

10 drops lemon oil

10 drops grapefruit oil

1. Put the baking soda in the Mason jar, with holes punched in the lid, so you can shake the freshener out onto the rug, or use a clean, empty salt canister, and add the essential oil drops. Cover the lid with your hand and shake well.

2. Sprinkle the powder on your carpet and allow it to sit on the carpet for about 30 minutes, then vacuum the powder from the carpet.

TIP: One great container for this mixture is an empty salt canister. Once you use all the salt, take out the metal spout, shake out as much of the salt as you can (and getting a little salt on your carpet won't hurt the fabric) and then use a funnel to get the carpet freshener into the canister.

Morning Bathroom Spray

My bathroom always seems to be damp and musty, even though I almost always keep the window open. My solution to this problem is to use this spray before I leave for work. It freshens the room and, when I come home eight hours later, the bathroom is a bit more welcoming than it would be without.

LEVEL: Easy

MAKES: 1 (8-ounce) spray bottle

Ingredients

4 ounces witch hazel

4 ounces distilled water

20 drops lemon essential oil

20 drops peppermint essential oil

20 drops tea tree essential oil

10 drops rosemary essential oil

10 drops sweet orange essential oil

Pour water and witch hazel into a spray bottle. Add the essential oils and gently shake to combine. Spray into air and allow to settle.

Romantic Dream Sachet

I can't promise you'll have sweet dreams if you put this sachet in one of your pillows, but I do know from experience that many of us experience anxious and repetitive thoughts—someone I once knew called it "cerebral nausea"—when we try to sleep. If you can focus on your deep breathing and the scent of this sachet, you may be able to release that unproductive thinking pattern.

LEVEL: Hard

MAKES: 1 sachet

Ingredients

4 x 8-inch piece of muslin

needle

thread

¼ cup dried lavender

½ cup flaxseeds

20 drops lavender essential oil

10 drops chamomile essential oil

10 drops lemon essential oil

1. Fold the muslin in half, so the outside faces inward.

2. Sew the two side ends together tightly and sew most of the top, leaving an inch or so open to put in the potpourri.

3. Mix the dried lavender, flaxseeds, and essential oils together in a small bowl, and add the mixture into the sachet using a spoon.

4. Tightly sew the rest of the sachet. Place in the bottom corner of one of your pillows, away from the opening.

White Fir Toilet Refresher

While others might tell you that you can use this without scrubbing, I'm not going to lie—you will need a toilet brush. But, this is a great item to put in the toilet before you use a toilet brush. You can use the long-handled toilet brush, which, to me, makes a big difference.

LEVEL: Hard

MAKES: 6 Easter egg-sized molds

Ingredients

½ cup baking soda

½ cup citric acid

½ cup borax

water, as needed

25 drops white fir essential oil

1. Add all dry ingredients to a small bowl and stir.

2. Adding a few drops of water at a time, stir until you have a crumbly mixture. You'll know the mixture is ready if you hold it in your hand and it keeps its shape. Add the essential oil and mix again.

3. Press the mixture into both halves of Easter egg molds, pressing out the air. Put a small bit of water on the tops of the molds before closing. Leave the molds dry for two days, then unmold.

4. Store in a glass jar with a tight fitting lid until ready to use.

5. To use: Drop one refresher into the toilet and wait for the fizzing to stop. Use a toilet brush to clean the toilet, then flush.

Lemon Vanilla Foyer Spray

I mention in other recipes that I sometimes try to mimic the scents created by fragrance companies, and this recipe is a direct result of that experimentation. I walked into Sephora one day and noticed that there was a new (at least to me) perfume company centered around the scent of vanilla, which, while common in foods, has just begun to be used in many fragrances. Paired with lemon, it is a perfect scent to welcome visitors to your home.

LEVEL: Easy

MAKES: 1 (8-ounce) spray bottle

Ingredients

3 ounces witch hazel

3 ounces water

20 drops lemon essential oil

20 drops vanilla essential oil

1. Add all ingredients to the spray bottle. Shake gently.

2. Spray a small bit of this toward a fan or near a vent and the scent will waft around the room. This is a concentrated scent, so you don't need to use a lot.

Warming Sleep Pillow

Like a puppy, my nose is always cold, and while this pillow is for your eyes, it is very soothing on a cold night.

LEVEL: Hard

MAKES: 1 pillow

Ingredients

sunglasses

piece of paper

pencil

½ yard fabric

thread

needle

1½ cups flaxseed

25 drops frankincense essential oil

25 drops cypress essential oil

1. To make the template for your pillow, put a pair of sunglasses on top of a piece of paper and trace around them, making your line about half an inch wider than the actual size of the glasses. You can make your design slightly more rectangular or circular than the shape of glasses, whatever you find more attractive.

2. Put the paper on the fabric, and cut a piece of fabric from the pattern. Repeat to create an identical pattern. One piece of fabric will be the front of the eye pillow and the second will be for the back.

3. Put the pieces of fabric on top of each other with the outside patterns facing inward. Pin them together and sew around the edges, leaving about ¼ inch of fabric as the seam. Leave one inch unsewn so that you will be able to fill it with flax. Then, flip your mask right side out.

4. Put the flaxseed in a bowl and add the drops of essential oil. Stir gently and thoroughly.

5. Funnel the flaxseed into the pillow.

6. Sew the hole closed tightly using a whipstitch.

7. If you want, you can make the eye pillow warm by microwaving for 10 seconds at a time in the microwave (remember that the middle gets hotter than the outside).

TIP: Because this is filled with food, I only keep these eye pillows for a few months at a time. If you want to refresh the scent, you can spritz it with a hydrosol and let it dry a bit before putting it on your eyes.

White Fir Holiday Candles

Most of the holidays and celebrations we have during winter honor light in some way, and, of course, that makes a lot of sense. Winter is a dark season and so we want to bring light into our lives.

LEVEL: Hard

MAKES: 6 (8-ounce) candles

Ingredients

25 drops white fir essential oil

15 drops bergamot essential oil

10 drops lemon essential oil

natural food coloring (optional)

6 Mason jars

6 cotton wicks

6 pencils

double boiler

3 pounds organic beeswax

1. Clean the Mason jars and dry them thoroughly.

2. Put water in the bottom of a double boiler, place the boiler on the stove, and turn on the heat until the water reaches a simmer.

3. Place beeswax in the top part of the boiler until it melts, about 5 minutes over low heat. Once it has melted, remove it from the heat and stir in the essential oils. Add food color, if using, one drop at a time, until desired color is achieved.

4. Cut the wicks to be twice the size of your clean Mason jars. Tape one end of each wick the middle of a pencil or stick, wrap the wick around the pencil a few times, and then let it hang over and into the jar.

5. Slowly pour the wax into the Mason jars so the wax covers the wick. Leave the wick in place and put the candle in a cool place. Cover lightly with a towel and let it harden for a day.

6. When the wax has hardened, cut the wick to the right length.

Diffuser Blends

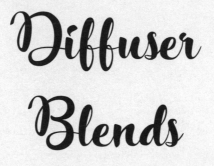

Lemon and Basil Room Freshener

This is the perfect kitchen freshener, especially if you've been cooking with a lot of oil. Sometimes excess oil can leave a rancid smell, and lemon and basil will help revive a kitchen. First, of course, open the window to let out the scent of oil, and use the lemon and basil to bring your kitchen back to life.

LEVEL: Easy

MAKES: 1 use

Ingredients

>   10 drops lemon essential oil

>   10 drops basil essential oil

Add essential oils to a diffuser. Follow diffuser directions.

TIP: Although this is a perfect scent for the kitchen, I would not spray this on surfaces, as the scent of food can be attractive to insects. In a diffuser, however, the scent is perfect and won't interfere with the scent of whatever you are cooking.

Five Floral and Energizing Diffuser Blends

Is there any better scent in the world than the flowers of spring. Lily-of-the-valley, lilac, and jasmine? Floral fragrances are romantic and pair nicely with the high energy that spring brings. To use these blends, follow the instructions on your diffuser.

LEVEL: Easy

MAKES: 1 use per blend

Blend #1

5 drops jasmine

3 drops peppermint

1 drop bergamot

Blend #2

5 drops ylang-ylang

5 drops sandalwood

5 drops lavender

Blend #3

5 drops ylang-ylang

5 drops clary sage

5 drops tangerine

Blend #4

5 drops geranium

5 drops spearmint

5 drops jasmine

Blend #5

5 drops blue tansy

5 drops helichrysum

5 drops lemon

Bergamot Hanging Car Diffuser

If you don't like the almost-chemical smell of most hanging air "fresheners," then this is the perfect project for you. It's also a wonderful gift. I've included a few of them in the book, as different scents work best in different seasons, and you can make your design fit the scent and the season. This recipe doesn't specify amounts, as you can make as many or as few as you want in whatever size you'd like, which would be determined by the amount of clay you have.

LEVEL: Hard

MAKES: varies

Ingredients

 terra cotta air-dry clay

 bottle of bergamot essential oil

1. Place the essential oil in a jar with a lid. Cover and set aside.

2. Cover the counter or table with wax paper. Use a rolling pin to roll out your clay until it is about 1/4 inch thick, making sure to get rid of all air bubbles.

3. Using a cookie cutter or craft knife, cut out the shape you want.

4. Using a chopstick, make a small hole at the top of your shape where you will put the ribbon to hang your diffuser. If you want, you can use a toothpick to further decorate your diffuser.

5. Allow your diffuser to dry for about two days, and, when it's dry, use fine sandpaper to smooth any rough edges.

6. Tie a ribbon or cord through your diffuser.

7. Hang your diffuser over your rear-view mirror. To use, put five drops of oil on the diffuser. If the diffuser gets wet with water, let it dry again for a day or two, and then you can use again.

Basil and Lime Car Diffuser

If you use your car to trek to the beach and the woods during summer, this is a wonderful diffuser to help your car remain both airy and lightly scented. This is a very impressive make-and-take project, and if I had a loyal group of customers who were ready to learn some more complicated projects, I might invite them over for a diffuser party. Because these diffusers require a long wait time, I suggest you make them at your house and then invite your customers to come back the next day (or in two days), during which time you will have unmolded and wrapped them.

LEVEL: Hard

MAKES: 1 diffuser

Ingredients

terra cotta air-dry clay

50 drops patchouli essential oil

50 drops geranium essential oil

1. Combine essential oils in a glass jar with a lid. Stir to combine. Cover and set aside.

2. Cover the counter or table with wax paper. Use a rolling pin to roll out your clay until it is about ¼ inch thick, making sure to get rid of all air bubbles.

3. Using a cookie cutter or craft knife, cut out the shape you want.

4. Using a chopstick, make a small hole at the top of your shape where you will put the ribbon to hang your diffuser. If you want, you can use a toothpick to decorate your diffuser further.

5. Allow your diffuser to dry for about two days, and, when it's dry, use fine sandpaper to smooth any rough edges.

6. Tie a ribbon or cord through your diffuser.

7. Hang your diffuser over your rear-view mirror. To use, put five drops of oil on the diffuser. If the diffuser gets wet with water, let it dry again for a day or two, and then you can use again.

Five Cooling Blends

For many of us, the smells of fresh cut grass and coconut-scented Coppertone suntan lotion immediately bring us to summer. These blends can be used near your air conditioner to scent the room. Use in your diffuser, following the diffuser instructions.

LEVEL: Easy

MAKES: 1 use per blend

Blend #1

5 drops lavender essential oil

5 drops wild orange essential oil

5 drops coconut oil essential oil

Blend #2

5 drops lime essential oil

5 drops cedarwood essential oil

5 drops vanilla essential oil

Blend #3

5 drops lemon essential oil

5 drops bergamot essential oil

5 drops vanilla essential oil

Blend #4

5 drops lemongrass essential oil

5 drops tangerine essential oil

Five Focusing Diffuser Blends

Fall is a season of contradictions because the start of school requires us to focus, while the oncoming cool weather may make us want to cuddle up and rest. These diffuser blends were created for afternoon homework sessions, but on page 55 we have cuddle-worthy scents! Use these blends in a diffuser, following your diffuser's instructions.

LEVEL: Easy

MAKES: 1 use per blend

Blend #1
5 drops basil essential oil

5 drops lavender essential oil

Blend #2
5 drops cypress essential oil

5 drops lemongrass essential oil

Blend #3
5 drops bergamot essential oil

5 drops black pepper essential oil

Blend #4
5 drops peppermint essential oil

5 drops grapefruit essential oil

Blend #5
5 drops tangerine essential oil

5 drops ginger essential oil

Tea Tree Oil and Lavender Hanging Car Diffuser

If your children play a lot of sports during the school year, this is a great item to keep in your car to take away the scent of equipment and sweaty clothes. This recipe doesn't specify amounts, as you can make as many or as few as you want in whatever size you'd like, which would be determined by the amount of clay you have.

LEVEL: Hard

MAKES: varies

Ingredients

 terra cotta air-dry clay

 50 drops tea tree essential oil

 50 drops lavender essential oil

1. Combine essential oils in a glass jar with a lid. Stir to combine. Cover and set aside.

2. Cover the counter or table with wax paper. Use a rolling pin to roll out your clay until it is about 1/4 inch thick, making sure to get rid of all air bubbles.

3. Using a cookie cutter or craft knife, cut out the shape you want.

4. Using a chopstick, make a small hole at the top of your shape where you will put the ribbon to hang your diffuser. If you want, you can use a toothpick to decorate your diffuser further.

5. Allow your diffuser to dry for about two days, and, when it's dry, use fine sandpaper to smooth any rough edges.

6. Tie a ribbon or cord through your diffuser.

7. Hang your diffuser over your rear-view mirror. To use, put five drops of oil on the diffuser. If the diffuser gets wet with water, let it dry again for a day or two, and then you can use again.

Eucalyptus and Orange Blossom Diffuser Stones

This is an inexpensive and impressive gift to make for friends and family, or for a make-and-take party. They are small and, when given with a small bottle of oil, they make very thoughtful hostess gifts, too. You can use any combination of oils.

LEVEL: Hard

MAKES: 12 small diffusers

Ingredients

2 cup baking soda

¾ cup water

50 drops eucalyptus essential oil

50 drops orange blossom essential oil

2 tablespoons grapeseed oil

1. Preheat oven to 400 degrees. Prepare a sheet of silicone molds.

2. Put the baking soda in the mixing bowl, and slowly add the water, because the mix needs to be drier than you would expect. Mix with a spoon, at first, but eventually you will need to use your hands to make sure the mix is moldable.

3. Put the mix into the molds, making sure to remove air bubbles.

4. Bake for 30 minutes.

5. Take the stones out of the mold and arrange them in a decorative bowl. When you want to scent your living room, just put some drops of your essential oil mix on the stones.

TIP: Because these are for fall and, in my mind, the living room, I would suggest using circle molds, but you can make these for Christmas and use candy cane or gingerbread men molds, or flower molds for spring, and pair with the right oils for the season.

Vanilla Sugar Car Diffuser

Using stamps to make patterns is a creative way to make diffusers for your car. You can buy sets of stamps to make a collection of related patterns, such as fall leaves or the initials of the people in your family. Use more clay to make as many diffusers as you'd like.

LEVEL: Hard

MAKES: varies

Ingredients

terra cotta air-dry clay

small bottle vanilla essential oil

natural food coloring (optional)

1. Combine essential oils in a glass jar with a lid. Stir to combine. Cover and set aside.

2. Cover the counter or table with wax paper. Use a rolling pin to roll out your clay until it is about 1/4 inch thick, making sure to get rid of all air bubbles. Add food coloring, if you'd like.

3. Using a cookie cutter or craft knife, cut out the shape you want.

4. Using a chopstick, make a small hole at the top of your shape where you will put the ribbon to hang your diffuser. If you want, you can use a toothpick to further decorate your diffuser.

5. Allow your diffuser to dry for about two days, and, when it's dry, use fine sandpaper to smooth any rough edges.

6. Tie a ribbon or cord through your diffuser.

7. Hang your diffuser over your rear-view mirror. To use, put five drops of oil on the diffuser. If the diffuser gets wet with water, let it dry again for a day or two, and then you can use again.

Five Cuddle-Worthy Diffuser Blends

Fireplaces. November rains. The chill in the air. Sometimes, in fall, you want to sit inside and relax with a book, play a board game with your kids, or snuggle with your honey. These scents will create an atmosphere of warmth and intimacy.

LEVEL: Easy

MAKES: 1 use per blend

Blend #1
5 drops rose essential oil

5 drops rosewood essential oil

Blend #2
5 drops ylang-ylang essential oil

5 drops lavender essential oil

Blend #3
5 drops clary sage essential oil

5 drops cardamom essential oil

Blend #4
5 drops patchouli essential oil

5 drops apple essential oil

Blend #5
5 drops cinnamon essential oil

5 drops clove essential oil

5 drops peppermint essential oil

White Fir Christmas Tree Diffuser

This is a lovely way to keep the scent of the holidays moving through your house. This recipe doesn't specify amounts, as you can make as many or as few as you want in whatever size you'd like, which would be determined by the amount of clay you have.

LEVEL: Hard

MAKES: 1 diffuser

Ingredients

terra cotta air-dry clay

bottle white fir essential oil

1. Cover the counter or table with wax paper. Use a rolling pin to roll out your clay until it is about 1/4 inch thick, making sure to get rid of all air bubbles.

2. Using a cookie cutter or craft knife, cut out the shape you want.

3. Using a chopstick, make a small hole at the top of your shape where you will put the ribbon to hang your diffuser. If you want, you can use a toothpick to decorate your diffuser further.

4. Allow your diffuser to dry for about two days, and, when it's dry, use fine sandpaper to smooth any rough edges.

5. Tie a ribbon or cord through your diffuser.

6. Hang your diffuser over your rear-view mirror. To use, put five drops of oil on the diffuser. If the diffuser gets wet with water, let it dry again for a day or two, and then you can use again.

Nutmeg and Cinnamon Car Diffuser

This is a perfect scent for winter months when you are traveling in your car for a long time. It is both warming and energizing. Cinnamon is remarkably beneficial to when you eat it, so stir the powder into your oatmeal on a cold winter morning.

LEVEL: Hard

MAKES: 1 diffuser

Ingredients

terra cotta air-dry clay

½ bottle nutmeg essential oil

½ bottle cinnamon essential oil

1. Combine essential oils in a glass jar with a lid. Stir to combine. Cover and set aside.

2. Cover the counter or table with wax paper. Use a rolling pin to roll out your clay until it is about 1/4 inch thick, making sure to get rid of all air bubbles.

3. Using a cookie cutter or craft knife, cut out the shape you want.

4. Using a chopstick, make a small hole at the top of your shape where you will put the ribbon to hang your diffuser. If you want, you can use a toothpick to further decorate your diffuser.

5. Allow your diffuser to dry for about two days, and, when it's dry, use fine sandpaper to smooth any rough edges.

6. Tie a ribbon or cord through your diffuser.

7. Hang your diffuser over your rear-view mirror. To use, put five drops of oil on the diffuser. If the diffuser gets wet with water, let it dry again for a day or two, and then you can use again.

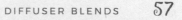

Vanilla and Cedarwood Hanging Car Diffuser

If your children play a lot of sports during the school year, this is a great item to keep in your car to take away the scent of equipment and sweaty clothes. This recipe doesn't specify amounts, as you can make as many or as few as you want in whatever size you'd like, which would be determined by the amount of clay you have.

LEVEL: Hard

MAKES: varies

Ingredients

terra cotta air-dry clay

50 drops vanilla essential oil

50 drops cedarwood essential oil

1. Combine essential oils in a glass jar with a lid. Stir to combine. Cover and set aside.

2. Cover the counter or table with wax paper. Use a rolling pin to roll out your clay until it is about 1/4 inch thick, making sure to get rid of all air bubbles.

3. Using a cookie cutter or craft knife, cut out the shape you want.

4. Using a chopstick, make a small hole at the top of your shape where you will put the ribbon to hang your diffuser. If you want, you can use a toothpick to decorate your diffuser further.

5. Allow your diffuser to dry for about two days, and, when it's dry, use fine sandpaper to smooth any rough edges.

6. Tie a ribbon or cord through your diffuser.

7. Hang your diffuser over your rear-view mirror. To use, put five drops of oil on the diffuser. If the diffuser gets wet with water, let it dry again for a day or two, and then you can use again.

Five Warming Diffuser Blends

These five blends work to set a welcoming scent for your home, and you may notice that they all feature citrus (foods that are in season) and fragrant winter trees or spices. Follow the instructions on your diffuser to use.

LEVEL: Easy

MAKES: 1 use per blend

Blend #1

5 drops grapefruit essential oil

5 drops fir essential oil

3 drops black pepper essential oil

Blend #2

5 drops lemon essential oil

5 drops frankincense essential oil

5 drops spruce essential oil

Blend #3

5 drops clove essential oil

5 drops white pine essential oil

5 drops wintergreen essential oil

Blend #4

5 drops cardamom essential oil

5 drops cedar essential oil

3 drops peppermint essential oil

Blend #5

5 drops sandalwood essential oil

5 drops nutmeg essential oil

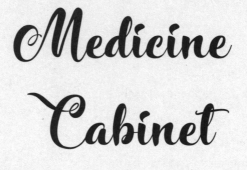

Medicine Cabinet

Eucalyptus and Camphor Anti-Allergy Inhaler

As a yoga teacher, I am all about the long, slow, deep breaths, and having colds drives me crazy because I can't stand not being able to breathe well. Few things are as healing and soothing to the stuffy nose as inhaling camphor. Remember Vicks VapoRub? VapoRub also uses camphor, but it is petroleum based, and no one needs fossil fuels on their bodies. This remedy is healthier and kinder to the planet. Because it is more of a self-treatment, it may not be best for a make-and-take party. This is also a wonderful recipe for a diffuser, although you may need to increase the amount of essential oil depending on the size of your diffuser.

LEVEL: Easy

MAKES: 1 inhaler

Ingredients

5 drops eucalyptus oil

5 drops camphor oil

hot water

1. Place very hot water in a large bowl on your kitchen counter. Don't put it on a table and, unless you are too sick, try to stand while you do this. Put the drops of oil in the bowl.

2. Bend over the bowl, tenting the towel over your head. As you inhale, bring the air down to your belly so you feel it expand, then continue to inhale, allowing the breath to fill your abdomen and then your chest. Consciously inhale as deeply as you can.

3. Exhale with intention, but not forcefully. Every few minutes, you may use an over-the-counter saline spray to clear your nasal passages.

Anti-Allergy Sleep Pillow

I have terrible spring allergies: pollen, trees, you name it. If it's outside, it makes my eyes burn. I love being outside, so I take allergy medicine, but I also use an eye pillow at night to soothe the burn. This pillow is for over your eyes, not for under your head. It's a great make-and-take for a class with kids if they want to learn to sew.

LEVEL: Hard

MAKES: 1 pillow

Ingredients

sunglasses

piece of paper

pencil

½ yard fabric

thread

needle

1 ½ cups flaxseed

20 drops frankincense essential oil

20 drops lemon essential oil

1. To make the template for your pillow, put a pair of sunglasses on top of a piece of paper and trace around them, making your line about half-inch wider than the actual size of the glasses. You can make your design slightly more rectangular or circular than the shape of glasses, whatever you find more attractive.

2. Put the paper on the fabric, and cut a piece of fabric from the pattern. Repeat to create an identical pattern. One piece of fabric will be the front of the eye pillow and the second will be for the back.

3. Put the pieces of fabric on top of each other with the outside patterns facing inward. Pin them together and sew around the edges, leaving about ¼ inch of fabric as the seam. Leave one inch unsewn so that you will be able to fill it with flax. Then, flip your mask right side out.

4. Put the flaxseed in a bowl and add the drops of essential oil. Stir gently and thoroughly.

5. Funnel the flaxseed into the pillow.

6. Sew the hole closed tightly using a whipstitch.

7. You can, if you want, make the eye pillow warm by microwaving for 10 seconds at a time in the microwave (remember that the middle gets hotter than the outside), or cool by putting it in the freezer for about 15 minutes.

TIP: Because this is filled with food, I only keep these eye pillows for a few months at a time. If you want to refresh the scent, you can spritz it with a hydrosol and let it dry a bit before putting it on your eyes.

Rosemary and Lavender Scalp Mask for Dandruff

Dandruff is very common and most people turn immediately to over-the-counter products. However, chemicals are not always the best solution for this type of problem because while they may temporarily fix the problem, they often have side effects or aren't actual re-balancing solutions. Natural remedies are better in the long term. In fact, the detergent-like recipes of most store-bought shampoos are not beneficial to the scalp or hair! If you suffer from dandruff, wash your hair at least every day, and, if necessary, twice a day. Stay away from processed foods, and eat plenty of vitamin-C rich foods.

LEVEL: Medium

MAKES: 1 (6-ounce) bottle

Ingredients

- 4 tablespoons argan oil
- 10 drops rosemary essential oil
- 10 drops lavender essential oil

1. In a small bowl, mix the oils together.

2. To use, massage oil into your scalp, using your fingertips and even, if it's comfortable, your fingernails (just a bit, you're not trying to scratch yourself, but to exfoliate the skin on your scalp a bit). You don't need to cover your hair, but make sure you don't just massage the top of your head, but the back and sides, too.

3. Cover your hair with a shower cap and leave it on your scalp for ten minutes.

4. Rinse, but don't shampoo. Do not go to sleep until your hair is dry and any residual oil is not coming off (you might need a towel to dry).

5. When you shampoo next, use an all-natural gentle clarifying shampoo without sulfates or other sudsing ingredients.

Geranium Antiperspirant

I love to sweat during my yoga classes, and while my sweat isn't typically stinky, I always want to err on the side of caution. After all, in my yoga classes, everyone is sweating, and the combination of everyone's body odor can be a lot. This antiperspirant helps with the kind of sweat that sometimes doesn't smell that good.

LEVEL: Easy

MAKES: 1 tube

Ingredients

¼ cup baking soda

¼ cup corn starch

2 tablespoons shea butter

15 drops geranium essential oil

15 drops tea tree essential oil

1. Stir baking soda, corn starch, shea butter, and essential oils in a small bowl.

2. Press the mixture into an empty deodorant tube and let rest in refrigerator for an hour so it solidifies more firmly.

3. Use as you would other antiperspirant.

Rollerball Foot Soother for Plantar Fasciitis

After a long hike or day at the beach, this roller bottle is like a massage for your feet. In fact, if you know anything about reflexology, you know that there are points on your feet that correspond to points on your body. According to the Mayo Clinic, "Reflexology is generally relaxing and may be an effective way to alleviate stress." Several studies show that reflexology may even help reduce pain, anxiety, and depression. Additionally, the essential oils in this rollerball provide significant health benefits. Wintergreen and clove have slight numbing effects, which can reduce the pain of plantar fasciitis, and lemongrass lowers inflammation. To me, this would make a great Father's Day gift. If you are having a make-and-take around that time, consider this as a project or giveaway for dads.

LEVEL: Easy

MAKES: 1 (50-milliliter) roller bottle

Ingredients

½ cup sweet almond oil

25 drops wintergreen essential oil

25 drops lemongrass essential oil

15 drops clove essential oil

1. Add all ingredients to a roller bottle and stir to combine.

2. To use, roll the ball under your foot and heel. If you are struggling with an acute case of plantar fasciitis, this is a nice way to massage your feet and strengthen the muscles of your lower legs.

Cooling Eyes Sleep Pillow

Sometimes, after a day at the beach in summer, my eyes burn from the sun, so I made this eye pillow to help my eye rest.

LEVEL: Hard

MAKES: 1 pillow

Ingredients

sunglasses

piece of paper

pencil

½ yard fabric

thread

needle

1 ½ cups flaxseed

25 drops peppermint essential oil

25 drops lavender essential oil

1. To make the template for your pillow, put a pair of sunglasses on top of a piece of paper and trace around them, making your line about half an inch wider than the actual size of the glasses. You can make your design slightly more rectangular or circular than the shape of glasses, whatever you find more attractive.

2. Put the paper on the fabric, and cut a piece of fabric from the pattern. Repeat to create an identical pattern. One piece of fabric will be the front of the eye pillow and the second will be for the back.

3. Put the pieces of fabric on top of each other with the outside patterns facing inward. Pin them together and sew around the edges, leaving about ¼ inch of fabric as the seam. Leave one inch unsewn so that you will be able to fill it with flax. Then, flip your mask right side out.

4. Put the flaxseed in a bowl and add the drops of essential oil. Stir gently and thoroughly.

5. Funnel the flaxseed into the pillow.

6. Sew the hole closed tightly using a whipstitch.

7. If you want, you can cool the pillow by putting it in the freezer for about 15 minutes.

TIP: Because this is filled with food, I only keep these eye pillows for a few months at a time. If you want to refresh the scent, you can spritz it with a hydrosol and let it dry a bit before putting it on your eyes.

After the Beach Cooling Spray

As with all make-and-takes, it's important that you only use this spray if you plan to be inside for at least a few hours. Essential oils can cause your skin to react negatively to UV rays, which is one reason there are no sunscreens in this book. I created this spray to help you cool off after a day in the sun.

LEVEL: Easy

MAKES: 1 (4-ounce) spray bottle

Ingredients

½ cup aloe vera gel

½ cup witch hazel

15 drops lavender essential oil

10 drops rose essential oil

1. Add all the ingredients to the glass bottle. Put the top on and shake gently.

2. Spray on your skin and let dry for a minute before sitting down. You can keep the bottle in the refrigerator to make it extra refreshing.

Motion Sickness Rollerball

The term "motion sickness" always reminds me of the great
Temptations song "Ball of Confusion," because it's a state of
being: your stomach is reacting to the mixed messages your body
is sending to your brain. Your inner ear may sense the feeling
of waves but your eyesight is leading your body so your body is
confused. Using essential oils will help you feel better, but it won't
change the symptoms. Instead, it may calm them and give your
senses something else to focus on altogether. Use the rollerball on
your wrists and temples, or just sniff it as needed.

LEVEL: Easy

MAKES: 1 small roller bottle

Ingredients

> 2 teaspoons sweet almond oil
>
> 5 drops ginger essential oil
>
> 5 drops lemongrass essential oil

Funnel the sweet almond oil into the roller bottle. Add the
essential oils, close the bottle, and shake gently to combine.

Lavender and Vitamin E Burn Salve

Between the grill, fireworks, and all the cooking and picnics in summer, small burns are bound to happen. I am not qualified to recommend medicines, but if you have a minor burn, these are traditional over-the-counter remedies, plus a little kick of essential oil. If you wanted to have a medicine chest make-and-take party, you could package these in washed lip gloss pots (which you can also buy new, but I am a big proponent of re-use and up-cycling packaging).

LEVEL: Easy

MAKES: 1 (4-ounce) glass bottle

Ingredients

¼ cup aloe vera gel

15 drops lavender essential oil

3 capsules vitamin E oil

1. Mix all ingredients in a bowl. I use a safety pin to poke a hole in the Vitamin E oil capsule and squeeze Vitamin E oil into the mix.

2. Put the salve on the burn. Cover it with a bandage or gauze.

Fennel and Mint Vertigo Relief

As people age, their inner ear changes and movement can cause vertigo or dizziness. The dizziness can be severe, but when it isn't overly bothersome, a centering blend of fennel and mint can help someone take deep breaths and get re-centered. You can use peppermint or spearmint, whichever you prefer. To use, apply the oil to the inside of your wrists or a cotton ball and inhale slowly.

LEVEL: Easy

MAKES: 1 small roller bottle

Ingredients

5 drops fennel essential oil

5 drops mint essential oil

2 teaspoons sweet almond oil

Funnel the oils into the roller ball bottle and close the bottle. Shake gently.

Lavender and Chamomile Soothe-the-Bite Oil

I am highly allergic to stings and bites. I stay swollen for weeks, and the first few days after a bite usually have me down for the count with fever and exhaustion. While this oil certainly can't fight the allergy, it relaxes my body (and my mind) from the stress of the bite. This mixture is for one application, but it can easily be quadrupled to fill a small bottle.

LEVEL: Easy

MAKES: 1 use

Ingredients

    1 teaspoon apple cider vinegar

    1 drop lavender essential oil

    1 drop chamomile essential oil

Mix all the ingredients in the bowl. Soak a cotton ball in the bowl, then apply to the site of the bite or sting.

Gingermint Upset Stomach Soother

I love mint tea. I drink it for relaxation, to help my stomach feel better after a big meal, and as a "dessert" in wintertime (it's so sweet, even without sugar, that it feels like dessert to me). This mixture will help settle a stomach upset by food or mood. Use your favorite mint essential oil—peppermint, spearmint, or wintergreen.

LEVEL: Easy

MAKES: 1 small roller bottle

Ingredients

2 tablespoons sweet almond oil

10 drops ginger essential oil

10 drops mint essential oil (peppermint, spearmint, or wintergreen)

1. Use a funnel to add all ingredients to a roller bottle. Shake gently to mix.

2. Roll on belly and on wrists to inhale the scent.

TIP: If you want to use this with younger children, decrease the amount of essential oil that you use and don't put it on their skin. Instead, have them either inhale from the rollerball or put the oil on a cotton ball that they can smell. Teach them to take deep breaths rather than sniff.

Tea Tree Clear Skin Drops

Tea Tree, which is a natural antibacterial, can help fight acne. Before using this, make sure your face is clean. This works well after using the Tea Tree Oil Face Wash.

LEVEL: Easy

MAKES: 1 small roller bottle

Ingredients

1 tablespoon aloe vera gel

15 drops tea tree oil

1 tablespoon apple cider vinegar

1. Pour all ingredients into a bowl and stir to combine. Funnel the mixture into a roller bottle and cover.

2. Use on pimples in the morning and before bed on a clean face.

Lavender Sleep Inducer

Lavender is all over this book, because it is one of the most effective essential oils, whether it is taken internally or used as a scent. Lavender is relaxing and helps reduce anxiety, and it helps people sleep better. It can help heal wounds and is an antioxidant. If someone were to ask me what essential oil to buy first, I would say lavender, and I would suggest using it at bedtime. You can simply add it to your bath, or you can spray it on your sheets, and that's what this make-and-take is: a spray for your sheets and pillow to help you sleep. I like lavender most when it is mixed with other essential oils so the scent is more complicated and interesting.

LEVEL: Easy

MAKES: 1 (4-ounce) spray bottle

Ingredients

25 drops lavender oil

10 drops lime oil

10 drops grapefruit oil

10 drops sweet orange oil

5 drops sweet basil oil

2 ounces witch hazel

10 tablespoons water

1. Pour all the ingredients into a jar and stir well. Then, funnel the mixture into a spray bottle.

2. To use, hold the spray bottle a few feet over your bed and spray, allowing the scent to fall onto your bed and pillows. You can also spray near your lamp, although not directly onto the light bulbs.

Screen-Time Recovery Sleep Pillow

These days, all of us look at screens too much. Besides taking breaks and looking at nature to rest your eyes, I try to go to bed at night without a screen near me. If my eyes are too tired to read a book, I simply use this eye pillow and listen to music to relax.

LEVEL: Hard

MAKES: 1 pillow

Ingredients

sunglasses

piece of paper

pencil

½ yard fabric

thread

needle

1 ½ cups flaxseed

25 drops helichrysm essential oil

25 drops cypress essential oil

1. To make the template for your pillow, put a pair of sunglasses on top of a piece of paper and trace around them, making your line about half an inch wider than the actual size of the glasses. You can make your design slightly more rectangular or circular than the shape of glasses, whatever you find more attractive.

2. Put the paper on the fabric, and cut a piece of fabric from the pattern. Repeat to create an identical pattern. One piece of fabric will be the front of the eye pillow and the second will be for the back.

3. Put the pieces of fabric on top of each other with the outside patterns facing inward. Pin them together and sew around the edges, leaving about ¼ inch of fabric as the seam. Leave one inch unsewn so that you will be able to fill it with flax. Then, flip your mask right side out.

4. Put the flaxseed in a bowl and add the drops of essential oil. Stir gently and thoroughly.

5. Funnel the flaxseed into the pillow.

6. Sew the hole closed tightly using a whipstitch.

7. You can, if you want, make the eye pillow warm by microwaving for 10 seconds at a time in the microwave (remember that the middle gets hotter than the outside), or cool by putting it in the freezer for about 15 minutes.

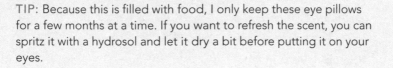

TIP: Because this is filled with food, I only keep these eye pillows for a few months at a time. If you want to refresh the scent, you can spritz it with a hydrosol and let it dry a bit before putting it on your eyes.

Geranium Mood Lifter

This is the essential oil mix I keep in my office. I don't want my office to smell like a spa, but I do want to have a scented space. I have this as a spray, but you could use the same blend in a candle or in a diffuser.

LEVEL: Easy

MAKES: 1 (8-ounce) spray bottle

Ingredients

3 ounces witch hazel

3 ounces distilled water

40 drops geranium essential oil

40 drops cedarwood essential oil

10 drops bergamot essential oil

10 drops ylang-ylang essential oil

5 drops peppermint essential oil

Pour water and witch hazel into a spray bottle. Add the essential oils and gently shake to combine. Spray into air and allow to settle.

Headache Ease Rollerball

I have an instinctual need to rub my head when I have a headache, and this rollerball helps with the self-massage. Plus, the essential oils will help to heal the pain. I suggest using the roller ball on the nape of your neck, as well as your temples.

LEVEL: Medium

MAKES: 1 small roller bottle

Ingredients

2 tablespoons grapeseed oil

20 drops peppermint essential oil

20 drops eucalyptus essential oil

10 drops lavender essential oil

5 drops rosemary essential oil

1. Add all ingredients to a bowl and stir gently to combine.

2. Funnel ingredients into a small roller bottle and secure the top. Apply to your forehead and temples.

Food Craving Control Blends

Scent contributes a great deal to our sense of hunger and satiety. Simply smelling food can make us hungry, but certain scents can also make us feel full. In a weight loss study, Dr. Alan Hirsch found that smelling peppermint can actually make you "feel" full and stop eating. Personally, I find that chewing gum or having a mint after a meal helps me. Because peppermint is sweet, it both feels like dessert and, according to Dr. Hirsch's research, affect's the brain satiety spot, the ventromedial nucleus of the hypothalamus.

I also find that citrus and rose scents, both of which also have a certain sweetness, help me feel full. In fact, two of my favorite things in the world are grapefruits (filling and delicious) and rose hip tea (delicious and good for the skin).

LEVEL: Easy

MAKES: 1 small dropper bottle each

Blend #1

30 drops peppermint essential oil

20 drops grapefruit essential oil

10 drops black pepper essential oil

Blend #2

30 drops rose essential oil

20 drops tangerine essential oil

10 drops bergamot essential oil

Add the essential oils to a small glass bottle and keep it nearby to inhale after a meal. If you are at a restaurant, I suggest heading outside for a moment to inhale. Even 30 seconds of mindful inhalation will help you during the dessert course.

Camphor and Wintergreen Muscle Soother

This oil will relax your muscles, whether you rub it in yourself or if you're lucky enough to have someone massage you with it.

LEVEL: Easy

MAKES: 1 (2-ounce) bottle

Ingredients

20 drops camphor essential oil

20 drops wintergreen essential oil

5 teaspoons sweet almond oil

1. Pour the sweet almond oil in the bowl, then add the drops of essential oils. Mix.

2. To use, place a towel underneath you, then massage the oil into the muscle that hurts (or have someone massage you with it). Be sure to wash your hands after using; this is an essential oil you don't want to get into your eyes.

Chamomile Heel Cream

Dancers are supposed to keep their heels and soles of the feet callused so that they don't get blisters from the floor and toes shoes, and I've found that as a yogi, I have a better grip on my mat when I don't moisturize my feet too much. But, I sometimes wake up in the middle of the night because my feet are so dry. (TMI? Sorry.) This cream makes a big difference in how my feet feel at night, but it's not designed to be used with a callus remover.

LEVEL: Hard

MAKES: 1 (12-ounce) bottle

Ingredients

¼ cup shea butter

¼ cup sweet almond oil

3 tablespoons beeswax

¼ cup castor oil

20 drops chamomile essential oil

water

1. Put a Mason jar in the top of the double boiler, and add about half a cup of water to the pot. Put on low heat, and add the shea butter, beeswax, and sweet almond oil to the top of the double boiler. Stir gently until melted.

2. Once the shea butter mixture has melted, turn off the heat, and pour the mixture into a bowl. Let it cool to room temperature. It will solidify.

3. Slowly add the chamomile oil, whisking to combine.

4. Store the jar in the refrigerator to maintain the consistency. When you want to use it, put it on your heels, and put on socks to keep the lotion on your feet without getting cream all over your floors.

Dry Scalp Soother

To use, move your hair in sections away from your scalp and point the spray bottle toward your scalp. Spray and then rub into your scalp with your fingertips. Use over your entire head. Sometimes it helps to gently (very gently!) scrub your scalp with your fingernails. You aren't trying to scratch yourself, but to exfoliate the dry skin away. Let the oil sit on your scalp for ten minutes and then rinse with a gentle shampoo, such as the Clary Sage Shampoo on page 96.

LEVEL: Easy

MAKES: 1 (4-ounce) glass bottle

Ingredients

¼ cup olive oil

10 drops lavender essential oil

10 drops rosemary essential oil

10 drops ho wood essential oil

glass spray bottle

Add all ingredients to a spray bottle and shake gently to mix.

Red Apple and Rose Callus Cream

As a dancer and yogi, my heels are always callused, and I have to balance my desire for smooth feet with my needs for calluses so that I don't slip on my yoga mat. When my feet are driving me crazy (frequently), I use a callus remover and this cream, and then I cover my feet with socks while the cream soaks in.

LEVEL: Hard

MAKES: 1 small Mason jar (about ½ cup)

Ingredients

4 tablespoons carnauba wax

1 tablespoon sweet almond oil

25 drops red apple oil

25 drops rose oil

25 drops chamomile oil

double boiler

wooden spoon

bowl

Mason jar

1. Put the wax and sweet almond oil in the top of the double boiler, with the water boiling over a low heat. Stir consistently.

2. Once mixed thoroughly, take the cream off the heat, and add the essential oils once it's a bit cool. Stir.

3. Put the cream into the Mason jar and cover with a clean towel while it cools completely. Then cover with the top of the jar.

4. Keep this cream in a cool place so that it remains thick and doesn't melt. When you put it on your feet, put on socks so that the cream doesn't get on your floors or furniture.

Tea Tree Toenail Antifungal

You can certainly use tea tree oil directly, but I thought I would create a recipe that includes other antifungal essential oils.

LEVEL: Easy

MAKES: 1 (1-ounce) dropper bottle

Ingredients

½ ounce tea tree essential oil

¼ ounce thyme essential oil

¼ ounce black pepper essential oil

Put all essential oils into a dropper bottle. To use, put the essential oil mixture on the toenail with the fungus. Do not cover, as darkness and moisture will encourage the growth of the fungus.

Clove and Lemon Warming Spray

I spend a lot of time in winter shoveling snow and ice from my long driveway, and when I come inside, my fingers and toes are cold and my body is hot (shoveling is a high calorie burner!). I use this spray to warm my extremities when I don't want to take a hot shower or bath.

LEVEL: Easy

MAKES: 1 (4-ounce) spray bottle

Ingredients

¼ cup sweet almond essential oil

10 drops clove essential oil

10 drops ginger essential oil

5 drops lemon essential oil

Add all ingredients to a glass bottle. When you come inside, spray a few drops of the oil into your hands and rub them into your feet, then cover with socks. Then, rub the oil into your hands and inhale.

Bath and Beauty

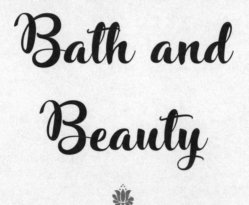

Geranium and Chamomile Hair Smoother

If your hair is frizzy, essential oils are a great way to smooth and shine the strands. Start with very little when you're first experimenting with their use to find the right amount for your hair's thickness. I think this is a great make-and-take gift for a spa or girl's-night-out party, especially if you live somewhere humid. Someone could spritz this on her hair and feel an immediate difference. To make it as a gift, pair it with a wooden comb.

LEVEL: Easy

MAKES: 1 (8-ounce) glass spray bottle

Ingredients

¼ cup water

1 tablespoon glycerin

5 to 20 drops geranium essential oil

5 to 20 drops chamomile essential oil

1. Using the funnel, add all ingredients to the spray bottle. Shake to mix.

2. Spray a small amount onto a hairbrush, and starting an inch or two away from your scalp, brush onto hair.

Rose and Tea Tree Skin Brightener Mask

We often feel more energetic and hopeful in spring, and your skin should reflect that youthful glow! This mask, especially if you pair it with a few minutes of meditation, will refresh you. For a bridal shower or spa make-and-take party, package the essential oils in a small bottle along with an unused mask in a small basket, or tie the mask to the bottle with a ribbon.

LEVEL: Medium

MAKES: 1 mask

Ingredients

2 tablespoons aloe vera gel

5 drops rose essential oil

5 drops tea tree essential oil

1. Combine the ingredients in a medium bowl.

2. Soak a pre-cut cloth mask in the bowl for about 30 seconds.

3. Take out the cloth and squeeze gently so it won't drip while on your face.

4. Put a towel on your bed and lie down, placing the mask on your face. Relax while for five minutes while wearing the mask.

TIP: You can buy mask cloths online. Typically, they are pieces of cotton or gauze cut in the shape of a face with eyeholes.

Clary Sage Hair Detangler

People with fine hair often need an extra rinse so that shampoo and conditioner won't weigh down their hair, but rinsing too often will leave fine hair tangled. Then, combing it can lead to breakage. This rinse will leave your hair shiny and easy to comb.

LEVEL: Hard

MAKES: 1 (16-ounce) glass bottle

Ingredients

2 tablespoons marshmallow root

1 cup water

1 tablespoon olive oil

20 drops clary sage essential oil

2 tablespoons apple cider vinegar

1. Add marshmallow root and water to a small pot and bring to boil, then reduce heat and simmer for 15 to 20 minutes. Remove from heat and cool.

2. Pour the marshmallow root mixture through a cheesecloth into a small bowl. In a separate bowl, add the essential oil and olive oil to the vinegar and allow to sit for a few minutes, then stir vigorously.

3. Add the marshmallow root mixture to the vinegar mixture and use a funnel to pour them into a spray bottle.

4. Shake well before using. Spritz onto dry or wet hair, let sit for 1–2 minutes, then comb through.

Flowering Bath Bomb

Bath bombs can be tricky to make, so, despite being impressive, they aren't great make-and-takes for your newer clients. However, if you have some return clients who might want to try a more complicated recipe together, or if you want to give someone a fancy gift, this would be perfect. This recipe assumes the molds are small, about 1 to 2 inches across.

LEVEL: Hard

MAKES: 12 small bath bombs

Ingredients

8 ounces baking soda

4 ounces Epsom salt

4 ounces corn starch

4 ounces citric acid

2 to 3 tablespoons castor oil

1 tablespoon water

15 drops neroli essential oil

10 drops helichrysum essential oil

natural food coloring (optional)

flower petals (optional)

1. In a large bowl, whisk together the baking soda, Epsom salt, corn starch, and citric acid. Keep a silicone mold with 12 forms nearby.

2. In a separate bowl, mix the castor oil, water, essential oils, and, food coloring, if using. Use only a single color of food coloring to guarantee that the bath water won't turn brown.

3. Very slowly, add the liquid to the dry mixture, whisking as you do so. The result should be a mixture that feels like damp sand.

4. Immediately put the mixture into the silicone molds, gently adding the flower petals to various parts of the mold. Press the mixture firmly into the molds before it begins to dry.

5. Cover the mold if you're using one that isn't ball/sphere-shaped and let the mixture dry for 24 hours.

Frankincense and Carrot Skin Serum

Like many vegetable essential oils, carrot seed oil smells earthy and is rich in antioxidants. It has been shown to repair cell damage caused by the sun, pollution, and other skin irritants.

LEVEL: Easy

MAKES: 1 (1-ounce) glass bottle

Ingredients

3 tablespoons avocado oil

10 drops frankincense essential oil

10 drops carrot seed essential oil

1. Pour the oils into a bowl and gently stir together.

2. Using a funnel, pour the oils into a small dark-colored glass dropper.

3. Use two to three drops of the oil on your face each night, allowing it to sink in before you get into bed.

Orange Facial Cleanser

Vitamin C is one of the best nutrients for your skin. It stimulates collagen production and is a strong antioxidant, so it fights the free radicals that age your skin and body.

LEVEL: Medium

MAKES: 1 (8-ounce) bottle

Ingredients

8 ounces unscented liquid Castile soap

zest of one orange

10 drops orange essential oil

1. Add the orange zest and the soap to a liquid measuring cup and stir gently. Add the essential oil.

2. Using the funnel, pour the mixture into the glass bottle.

3. When ready to use, put about a tablespoon in your hand, add water, and wash your face. Rinse thoroughly.

Clary Sage Shampoo and Conditioner for All Hair Types

This conditioner will do two important things: clean your scalp and condition your hair. Definitely use your fingertips to scrub your scalp while the shampoo/conditioner penetrates your ends. For different hair types, replace the clary sage and cedarwood with the combinations suggested below.

LEVEL: Medium

MAKES: 1 (8-ounce) bottle

Ingredients

one small avocado

two tablespoons honey

½ cup aloe vera juice

2 drops cedarwood essential oil

2 drops clary sage essential oil

1. Remove the peel and pit of the avocado, and mash or blend the avocado with the honey and aloe vera juice in a liquid measuring cup.

2. Add the essential oil combination that work for your hair type (see below).

3. Cover your head with the mixture and lather. Leave on for about 10 minutes, then rinse.

Essential Oil combinations for different hair types:

Oily hair: basil, eucalyptus, lemongrass

Fine hair: chamomile

Balance scalp dryness/oil: cedarwood

All hair types: clary sage

Dandruff: lemon, bitter orange

Floral Shower Sugar Scrub

I'm a scrub devotee because they make you feel clean and help slough away the outer layer of your skin. Plus, they prepare your body for lotion, which makes your skin even softer! If you want to make this a gift, I suggest tying a silk flower onto the bottle.

LEVEL: Easy

MAKES: 1 (16-ounce) Mason jar

Ingredients

1 cup turbinado sugar

½ cup avocado oil

1 tablespoon vitamin E oil

20 drops ylang-ylang essential oil

20 drops jasmine essential oil

10 drops tea tree essential oil

1. Pour all the ingredients in the measuring cup and mix.

2. Pour into short wide-mouth Mason jar and cover.

3. While in the shower, be sure to put the Mason jar where water will not hit it.

4. With your finger, take out some of the scrub, and use it on your body, being sure to rinse and not scrub very hard.

TIP: If your tub or shower feels greasy afterward, use the Grapefruit and Geranium Shower Spray on page 34. It will get rid of the residue from the enamel and tile.

Energizing Bubble Bath

Obviously, you could use detergent to get lots of bubbles, but let's face it, you really don't want to put detergent on your skin. The secret to the bubbles in this recipe is the egg whites. This recipe is for a single bath, and I included it because it can be a clever and fun gift. I love the idea of making a gift package with a small carton of egg whites, a teeny whisk, an eight-ounce bottle of soap, and a small bottle of mixed essential oils. How cute!

LEVEL: Medium

MAKES: 1 bath

Ingredients

3 egg whites

½ cup liquid Castile soap

10 drops orange essential oil

10 drops basil essential oil

1. Put egg whites in a liquid measuring cup and add soap and essential oils. Stir to combine.

2. While your bath water is running and when the tub is almost filled, start to pour the bubble bath slowly under the running water. Shut off the water soon after you've done this so that the extra water doesn't break all the bubbles.

TIP: Need some ideas for your leftover egg yolks? First, mixing the yolks with a few drops of rosemary essential oil and using it on your hair to condition. If you're hungry, extra egg yolks are often needed for puddings and can be mixed into a number of soups or pasta dishes.

No-Stress Lavender and Eucalyptus Bath Salts

Lavender and eucalyptus are two of my favorite scents. They are both calming and they remind me of some of my favorite places and memories. I don't make large amount of bath salts at once, as I find they don't stay dry enough in my bathroom, so this mixture is only good for one bath. If you want, though, you can double or triple this recipe and keep it in a closed Mason jar and use a handful or two when you take a bath.

LEVEL: Easy

MAKES: 1 large Mason jar

Ingredients

2 cups Epsom salt

¼ cup baking soda

5 tablespoons Dead Sea salts

2 tablespoons avocado oil

10 drops lavender essential oil

10 drops eucalyptus essential oil

1. Mix all ingredients in a small bowl.

2. Pour mixture into a wide-mouth Mason jar and close. Let it sit for a few hours before using, then add to your bath water when it's almost done filling the tub.

Rosemary and Cedarwood Split-End Spray

I try not to dissect people by their looks, but I do notice split ends because they are so easily fixed by a trim. A trim makes everyone's hair look better and doesn't noticeably change the length. If you are between trims, or if your hair needs some smoothing, this spray will help.

LEVEL: Easy

MAKES: 1 (1-ounce) spray bottle

Ingredients

15 drops rosemary essential oil

15 drops cedarwood essential oil

1 teaspoon apricot kernel oil

1 teaspoon water

Add all ingredients to a spray bottle and shake gently just before you use. Spray on the ends of wet hair, making sure not to use too much, as you don't them to look greasy. You can run your fingers through your hair or comb to make sure your hair has movement when it dries.

Lemon and Peppermint Hair Thickener

Experiencing the thinning of your hair is upsetting for both men and women. Cutting out simple sugars, such as cakes and candies, and eating a diet rich in Omega-3s can positively affect the health of your hair. Castor oil, or Ricinus communis, is a natural nutrient-rich food and beauty aid rich in ricinoleic acid, omega-6 and 9 fatty acids, vitamin E, and minerals. It is also a humectant, so it can help keep moisture in the hair shaft and scalp. Finally, because it is rich in antioxidants, it strengthens the keratin in the hair and can strengthen it while cutting down on frizz.

Of course, adding oil to your hair is not something you'll want to do before you go out. Instead, this should be a project for a spa night or to use while you soak in a hot tub. This recipe is for your scalp, but if you have long hair or want to use it on your hair, just double the recipe.

LEVEL: Easy

MAKES: 1 (4-ounce) dropper bottle

Ingredients

3 tablespoons castor oil

2 tablespoon olive oil

15 drops lemongrass essential oil

1. Add the liquids into a bottle with a narrow lid, such as a hair coloring bottle. Close the top with your finger and shake.

2. Separate sections of your hair and apply the oil to your scalp in sections. Cover your entire head with the oil. If there's extra oil, or if your hair is thick, you can comb the oil down to cover your hair.

3. Once the oil has been applied, massage your scalp to get the blood flowing.

4. You can cover your head with a towel to keep it warm and prevent the oil from getting on everything. Leave the oil on your scalp for 15 minutes.

5. Rinse your hair and, if you want, use a shampoo that cuts oil (such as one with tea tree) to get the oil out of hair.

Cornflower Oil Makeup Remover

Before you try this, make sure you understand that your eyes are sensitive and you should be careful about using any homemade product near your eyes. If you do some research online, you'll read that cornflower is widely used as an eye drop to help swollen and itchy eyes, and to reduce the irritation of sties and conjunctivitis. Nevertheless, start with a small amount of cornflower essential oil to make sure it doesn't irritate you.

LEVEL: Easy

MAKES: 20 makeup remover pads

Ingredients

2 tablespoons olive oil

2 tablespoons distilled water

4 drops cornflower essential oil

20 cotton pads

1. Pour the olive oil and water into a bowl and stir. Add the essential oil and mix gently.

2. Put the cotton pads into a Mason jar with a lid and pour the liquid over the pads.

3. Tightly put the lid on the jar and gently shake to distribute the liquid over the pads.

4. When you're ready to use, take out one pad, and gently wipe your eye makeup away.

Rosemary and Lavender Eyelash Serum

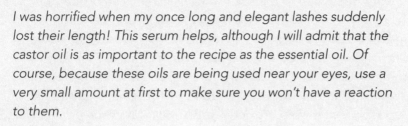

I was horrified when my once long and elegant lashes suddenly lost their length! This serum helps, although I will admit that the castor oil is as important to the recipe as the essential oil. Of course, because these oils are being used near your eyes, use a very small amount at first to make sure you won't have a reaction to them.

LEVEL: Easy

MAKES: 1 (1-ounce) dropper bottle

Ingredients

- ½ teaspoon castor oil
- 1 drop rosemary essential oil
- 1 drop lavender essential oil

1. Put the castor oil and essential oils in a glass dropper bottle and shake gently.

2. To use, after you wash your face at night, open the serum bottle and take a clean mascara brush. Dip it in the bottle and use as you would mascara. You can use this in the morning, but wait for it to dry before putting on your regular mascara.

Tomato Leaf Lip Balm

This project combines three of my favorite things: the scent of tomato, sunscreen, and lip balm. I've heard you can become addicted to lip balm, but I think that is only if you use the kinds with petroleum, which don't, in fact, lock moisture into your skin, but instead dries it out. This lip balm will truly make your lips softer and protect your lips from the sun, and it smells perfect for a summer make-and-take party! You can also give these as a gift to your guests. Add zinc oxide if you want a kick of sun protection, but it will change the color on your lips, and I can't guarantee the exact sun protection factor (SPF).

LEVEL: Hard

MAKES: 1 tube

Ingredients

3 teaspoons grated beeswax

5 teaspoons jojoba oil

½ teaspoon honey

6 drops tomato leaf essential oil

¼ teaspoon zinc oxide powder (optional)

1. Over a low heat, melt the beeswax and jojoba oil in a double boiler, stirring to mix fully.

2. Remove from the heat, and stir in honey and essential oil. Once thoroughly mixed, add the zinc oxide powder, if using, until it is thoroughly mixed in.

3. Pour into empty lip balm containers (you can use an old one that you have wash and dried thoroughly). Let set for 30 minutes before moving or covering.

TIP: If you want to add a small bit of color, you can melt a tiny amount of an old lipstick into the mixture during the first step. Don't add too much or the mixture will become too thick.

Scrunchy Beachy Hair Spray

I have thin, fine hair, and it tends to lie flat, but this spray allows me to boost it with a little texture. I wouldn't recommend it for people with naturally wavy hair, as it will make it brittle. This will create a very wet look, especially if your hair is thin (you may need less). This is a great project for a vacation-themed make-and-bake party for reliable customers who are looking for more elaborate recipes.

LEVEL: Medium

MAKES: 1 (8-ounce) spray bottle

Ingredients

hot water

¼ cup Epsom salts

¼ cup sea salt

1 tablespoon aloe vera gel

1 tablespoon unscented base conditioner (see note)

10 drops orange essential oil

10 drops lavender essential oil

1. Put hot water in a large bowl and add the Epsom salts, sea salt, aloe vera, conditioner, and essential oils. Mix well.

2. Pour the mixture into a glass spray bottle using the funnel, then gently shake.

3. Wash your hair at night and spray with the mixture. Braid or twist your hair while it's damp and spray again. Cover with a shower cap and sleep. In the morning, take off the cap and untwist. Don't brush! Use your fingers or a wide-tooth comb to separate strands.

TIP: You can buy bulk conditioners from online apothecaries, or look in your local natural food store for unscented conditioner. You can use this as your base conditioner.

Lemon and Lavender Oily Hair Spray

Sometimes oily hair is due to an overproduction of hormones and sometimes it is a reaction to the drying ingredients of most consumer hair products. Washing your hair with gentle shampoo and brushing it regularly will help, as well using essential oils that balance the production of scalp oils. I recommend using this at night.

LEVEL: Easy

MAKES: 1 (eight-ounce) spray bottle

Ingredients

3 ounces witch hazel

3 ounces distilled water

10 drops lemon oil

10 drops lavender oil

10 drops cedarwood essential oil

1. Add all ingredients to a glass spray bottle and shake gently.

2. Spray on your roots and then use a brush to spread it through your hair. I suggest that you only use a little bit at first to see how your hair feels in the morning.

Geranium Hair Detangler Spray

My hair is long and fine, and it tangles the most when it's in need of a trim. Long hair and fine hair, and especially the hair of a young child, are most likely to tangle. The best thing to do to avoid tangles is comb your hair frequently, and if you're going to be active, use a coated rubber band to keep your healthy and untangled. You can use this spray sparingly before you comb in the morning and then, at night, after a shower. I think it works best on wet hair. Unless your hair is very thick, dry, and flyaway, I don't think it is best to use essential oils during the day.

LEVEL: Medium

MAKES: 1 (4-ounce) spray bottle

Ingredients

3 tablespoons olive oil

3 tablespoons avocado oil

1 tablespoon shea butter

10 drops geranium essential oil

10 drops sandalwood essential oil

1. Mix all ingredients in a bowl, then funnel them into a glass spray bottle.

2. Keeping the bottle at least an inch or two away from your head, spray the oils onto your hair in sections, combing through as you go.

3. Fluff your hair with your fingers when done to distribute the oils further.

Clary Sage Deep Conditioner

I am a big believer in hair conditioner, even though my hair is fine and thin. It's true, I don't use heavy conditioners, but I do make my hair silky and shiny with this conditioner. It's a great product to use once a week. If your hair is thick and course, you can use Shea butter with rosemary, ylang-ylang, and myrrh essential oils. This recipe will make a bottle that should last through four or five uses.

LEVEL: Medium

MAKES: 1 (4-ounce) bottle

Ingredients

5 tablespoons sweet almond oil

2 tablespoons jojoba oil

10 drops lavender essential oil

10 drops clary sage essential oil

10 drops geranium essential oils

1. Put all ingredients in mixing bowl and whisk to bring some air into the mixture. Transfer ingredients to a bottle.

2. To use, apply to the strands of your hair in the shower. Comb through to distribute.

3. Get out of the shower and sit with the conditioner on your hair for 15 minutes.

4. Get back in shower and rinse. If you need to shampoo for the day, use a gentle all-natural shampoo without sulfates or other chemicals that will strip your hair of its oils.

Festival Hand Lotion

I call this festival hand lotion because the patchouli reminds me of music festivals. It is very light and won't sit on your skin and make it greasy. This is how I usually use lotion and oil: After I shower or wash my hands, I put lotion or oil on, let it dry a minute, and then wipe off the excess. Lotions and oils are designed to hold in moisture, so the most effective time to use them is after you bathe. However, if you're bringing this to a festival, I suggest you put some of what you make in an empty, clean lip gloss or blush pot to use when you aren't home. This would be a great make-and-take gift for more advanced essential oil fans.

LEVEL: Hard

MAKES: 1 (8-ounce) jar or tube

Ingredients

¼ cup shea butter

¼ cup fractionated coconut oil

15 drops patchouli essential oil

15 drops palmarosa essential oil

1. Heat the shea butter and coconut oil in a double boiler over a low to medium flame until they are liquid and combined.

2. Remove the mixture from the heat, put it in a glass bowl, and put in refrigerator for a half hour.

3. Remove from the refrigerator, add the essential oils, and use a hand mixer to add air to the mixture.

4. Put the mixture in a Mason jar, and when you want to use, take a nickel-sized amount, simply rub in your hands. When not using, cover with a lid.

Cooling Spearmint Bath Bomb

I do not like hot weather and so frequently, after a summer day, I take a cool bath or a cool shower before I go to sleep. Bath bombs are great gifts, although they take a little more work than other projects. This is a perfect hostess gift for your customers to make and give to friends and family, but you can also give them to your customers when they come to a make-and-take party. Be sure to wrap them with the recipe.

LEVEL: Hard

MAKES: 12 small bath bombs

Ingredients

½ cup baking soda

½ cup citric acid

½ cup borax

water

10 drops spearmint essential oil

10 drops lemongrass essential oil

plastic molds

1. In a large bowl, whisk together the baking soda, Epsom salt, corn starch, and citric acid. Keep a silicone mold with 12 forms nearby.

2. In a separate bowl, mix the castor oil, water, essential oils, and, food coloring, if using. Use only a single color of food coloring to guarantee that the bath water won't turn brown.

3. Very slowly, add the liquid to the dry mixture, whisking as you do so. The result should be a mixture that feels like damp sand.

4. Immediately put the mixture into the silicone molds. Press the mixture firmly into the molds before it begins to dry.

5. Cover the mold if you're using one that isn't ball/sphere-shaped and let the mixture dry for 24 hours.

Lavender and Ylang-Ylang Cuticle Cream

I love getting manicures, but I often can't find the time! I've come to realize that pushing back my cuticles on my own is easy and takes very little time. This cream, paired with a cuticle stick, will help your nails stay healthy. I even use it on my toenails. And, honestly, this rich cream feels great on heels, too.

LEVEL: Easy

MAKES: 1 small wide-mouthed Mason jar

Ingredients

5 tablespoons organic beeswax

3 tablespoons organic raw shea butter

1 tablespoon organic coconut oil

5 drops vitamin E oil

15 drops lavender essential oil

10 drops ylang-ylang essential oil

5 drops tea tree essential oil

1. Mix all ingredients in a bowl, then put into a small glass jar.

2. When ready to use, spoon out the cream and use one finger of your other hand to massage into your cuticles. Gently push them back with your finger or a cuticle stick.

Witch Hazel and Rose Facial Toner

If you spend the day swimming, whether in a pool, lake, or the ocean, this is a great solution to having salt water or chlorine residue on your skin. It's gentle, and rose is wonderful for the health of your skin. In fact, there are a number of fancy (and expensive!) rose beauty products that either have rose petals in them or rose oil. Buying rose essential oil and making your own toner is exactly the same as what you can buy, only much less expensive.

LEVEL: Easy

MAKES: 1 (4-ounce) bottle

Ingredients

½ cup witch hazel

20 drops rose essential oil

20 drops tea tree essential oil

1. Pour the witch hazel into a glass bottle with a lid, and add all ingredients. Gently shake to combine.

2. Pour a small amount onto a cotton ball and use all over clean face.

Cooling Summer Sugar Scrub

When I come inside at the end of the day, I take off my shoes, put my things down, and wash my hands, but I dislike using soap, as it is often drying. This is a better choice, as it exfoliates a bit and the oils are cooling, which feels lovely on a hot day. This recipe makes one use, so you could package it as a gift for a make-and-take party, or you could use it as a sample project for your guests.

LEVEL: Easy

MAKES: 1 use

Ingredients

2 tablespoons brown sugar

1 tablespoon olive oil

10 drops vanilla essential oil

5 drops tea tree essential oil

Mix all ingredients in a small bowl. Rub on your hands and "wash" with the scrub. Be gentle and rinse well.

No-Ouch Bikini Shave Lotion

Many women feel that shaving is the most effective way to get rid of upper thigh hair. When shaving this area, use a very sharp (new) razor, and use this lotion, which will soften the hair. Oils, by the way, dull razors, which is why this recipe is more lotion than oil. Make sure you shave after being in the shower for at least a few minutes, too.

LEVEL: Hard

MAKES: 1 (12-ounce) bottle

Ingredients

¼ cup jojoba oil

¼ cup shea butter

½ cup grapeseed oil

10 drops calendula essential oil

10 drops chamomile essential oil

1. Using a double boiler, melt the shea butter. Add the jojoba and grapeseed oils while slowly stirring.

2. Remove from the heat and cover. Put it in the refrigerator for about 45 minutes to chill. The mixture will not harden.

3. Using a hand mixer, whip the lotion to add air and make it lighter. Stir in the neroli oil, then use a spoon or spatula to scoop into a small wide-mouth Mason jar. Cover until ready to use.

Chamomile and Carrot Seed Split End Spray

Both chamomile and carrot seed are wonderful for split ends because they nourish the strands as they protect the hair, too. Split ends are a sign that you aren't treating your hair well. Brushing wet hair and using blow dryers both weaken and damage hair, and so does using a lot of chemical hair product, which removes the natural oils from hair. Using essential oils on your hair are like eating a salad instead of a sandwich with processed meat and bread: it's healthy and enriching. Simply spray this mixture onto the ends of your hair and massage it into the strands.

LEVEL: Medium

MAKES: 1 (1-ounce) bottle

Ingredients

10 drops chamomile essential oil

10 drops carrot seed essential oil

3 tablespoons argan oil

Mix all oils in bowl, then funnel the oils into a spray bottle.

Black Currant Oil Facial Scrub

Not used frequently because its fragrance is neither floral nor woodsy, black currant oil is high in gamma linolenic acid, an essential fatty acid that's good for your skin! Also, I've always been a fan of using baking soda as a gentle scrub. I make this in one-dose batches to use before bed or in the shower. If you want, you can use an essential oil serum after this, such as the Frankincense and Carrot Skin Serum (page 94).

LEVEL: Easy

MAKES: 1 use

Ingredients

3 tablespoons baking soda

5 drops black currant essential oil

1. Put baking soda in bowl and add drops of essential oil.

2. Using a very gentle circular motion, wash face with mixture. Rinse well.

Moisturizing Hand Sugar Scrub

I created this recipe one night when I looked down at my hands and thought everything about them looked old and unkempt. I decided to take ten minutes to take care of them. My solution included cutting my nails, pushing back my cuticles (see Lavender and Ylang-Ylang Cuticle Cream on page 113) and using this scrub. Not only did I go to bed feeling a little bit prettier, but I specifically used essential oils with a scent that would relax me.

LEVEL: Easy

MAKES: 1 use

Ingredients

2 tablespoons brown sugar · 10 drops vanilla essential oil

1 tablespoon olive oil · 5 drops tea tree essential oil

Mix all ingredients in a medium bowl. To use, rub the scrub on your hands. Be gentle and rinse well.

Epsom Salt Spa Bath

Soaking (or swimming) in salt water is one of the best things we can do for our bodies and our spirits. If you're not near the ocean, then a salt water bath should be one of your weekly habits. It's inexpensive and, especially if you're very active, wonderful for helping the body to recover from intense workouts.

LEVEL: Easy

MAKES: 1 bath

Ingredients

2 cups Epsom salt

¼ cup sweet almond oil

10 drops lavender essential oil

10 drops eucalyptus essential oil

Pour all ingredients into a Mason jar and mix. To use, pour ¼ cup into bath as the water runs.

TIP: This is a wonderful make-and-take to pair with a little spoon, ribbon, recipe, and directions for use in your guests' homes.

Muscle-Soothing Bubble Bath

When I was in yoga teacher training, it was not uncommon for us to do four hours of yoga in one day. Of course, yoga is typically relaxing for your body, mind, and spirit, but four hours is a lot of work! At the end of the day, I would come home and soak in a tub using this mixture of oils. Heaven! Each of these oils has been shown to fight inflammation and help circulation. Plus, I would be ready for a second weekend of four more hours of yoga! You can pre-mix this bath and put the mixture in individual bottles to give as gifts to the athletes in your life.

LEVEL: Easy

MAKES: 1 bath

Ingredients

    10 drops wintergreen essential oil

    10 drops basil essential oil

    10 drops sweet marjoram

Add the essential oils straight to your tub.

Palmarosa Moisturizing Facial Mask

Dry skin is a problem for many women, especially women who are post-menopause. Drinking water will help. It's also important to care for your skin to hold in moisture. Also, it is helpful to eat healthy fats such as avocado, fish, nuts, and seeds. While oil and water don't mix outside of your body, you can use oils to keep the moisture from leaving your skin.

LEVEL: Hard

MAKES: 1 mask

Ingredients

5 drops palmarosa essential oil

5 drops sweet orange essential oil

5 drops chamomile essential oil

5 drops carrot seed essential oil

2 tablespoons avocado oil

1. Combine all ingredients in a medium bowl.

2. Soak a pre-cut cloth facial mask in the bowl for about 30 seconds.

3. Take out the cloth and squeeze gently so it won't drip while on your face.

4. Put a towel on your bed and lie down, placing the mask on your face. Relax for five minutes.

TIP: You can buy cloth masks with eyeholes online. They are pieces of cotton or gauze cut in the shape of a face.

Rosemary Lip Scrub

If your lips sometimes peel, it's usually due to dry skin. You can use lip balm, but gently removing the dry skin also helps. When you get out of the shower, you can use your towel and gently scrub your lips, then apply lip balm (especially the Tomato Leaf Lip Balm on page 106; don't use petroleum-based lip balm) to seal in the moisture. Don't scrub your lips more than once a week as the skin is very sensitive.

LEVEL: Easy

MAKES: 1 lip gloss pot

Ingredients

1 teaspoon brown sugar

1 teaspoon honey

1 teaspoon olive oil

1 to 2 drops rosemary essential oil

Combine all ingredients in a small glass bowl. To use, gently rub the mixture onto your lips in a circular motion, and then wipe or rinse off. Store in an airtight container.

Eucalyptus and Clary Sage Bath Bomb

A great project to make as a bridal shower giveaway, this recipe makes about a dozen bath bombs, though the exact number depends on the size of your silicone mold. You can also make this recipe with orange and spearmint, clary sage and rosemary, or rose and lavender.

LEVEL: Hard

MAKES: 12 small bath bombs

Ingredients

8 ounces baking soda

4 ounces Epsom salt

4 ounces corn starch

4 ounces citric acid

2 to 3 tablespoons castor oil

1 tablespoon water

1 to 2 teaspoons eucalyptus essential oil

1 to 2 teaspoons clary sage essential oil

natural food coloring (optional)

1. In a large bowl, whisk together the baking soda, Epsom salt, corn starch, and citric acid. Keep a silicone mold with 12 forms nearby.

2. In a separate bowl, mix the castor oil, water, essential oils, and, food coloring, if using. Use only a single color of food coloring to guarantee that the bath water won't turn brown.

3. Very slowly, add the liquid to the dry mixture, whisking as you do so. The result should be a mixture that feels like damp sand.

4. Immediately put the mixture into the silicone molds. Press the mixture firmly into the molds before it begins to dry.

5. Cover the mold if you're using one that isn't ball/sphere-shaped and let the mixture dry for 24 hours.

TIP: Add the wet to the dry mixture slowly so that the fizzing doesn't start before the bomb hits the bath.

Camphor and Eucalyptus Calming Bubble Bath

Being sick in winter cannot only feel bad physically, but it can also make you anxious. You're missing work and often can't breathe easily, both of which are very stressful. This bubble bath will relieve all of these symptoms.

LEVEL: Easy

MAKES: 1 bath

Ingredients

½ cup castile soap

10 drops camphor essential oil

10 drops eucalyptus essential oil

5 drops lavender essential oil

As the water is running and the tub is almost filled, pour the ingredients under the running water.

Neroli Body Soufflé

If you like body lotions that are lighter than air, this comes close! Designed not to clog your skin or feel too heavy, Body Soufflé is perfect for morning or before an evening out, and the scent is romantic.

LEVEL: Hard

MAKES: 1 Mason jar

Ingredients

⅓ cup shea butter

⅓ cup jojoba oil

3 cup grapeseed essential oil

10 drops neroli essential oil

1. Using the double boiler, melt the Shea butter. Add the jojoba and grapeseed oils while slowly stirring.

2. Remove from the heat and cover. Put it in the refrigerator for about 45 minutes. It can't harden, only chill.

3. Using a hand mixer, whip the lotion to add air and make it lighter. Stir in the neroli oil, then scoop into the Mason jar. Cover.

Other Recipes:

Rose and apple

Vanilla and bergamot

Moisturizing Red Apple and Rose Intensive Hand Cream

Years ago, I bought a relatively expensive hand cream because I was intoxicated by the aroma. I looked online and found that the main scents in the cream were apple, rose, and bergamot. I became intrigued and began to mix these essential oils in various measurements and products to create my own lotions. Thus, my passion was born.

LEVEL: Hard

MAKES: 1 (8-ounce) Mason jar

Ingredients

½ cup cold pressed coconut oil

½ cup olive oil

2 tablespoons beeswax pastilles

5 drops lavender oil

5 drops rose oil

1 tablespoon vitamin E oil

1. With water boiling in the double boiler, be sure the stove heat is on low, and add coconut oil, olive oil, and beeswax together; stir consistently.

2. Once brought together, bring off the heat, and stir in essential oil and vitamin E oil.

3. Spoon the lotion into the Mason jars, and let cool, covering with a kitchen towel as they cool.

4. Once cool, tighten the tops of the jar. If you live somewhere warm, I would keep this salve in the refrigerator so that it remains solid. You might want to keep a small wooden spoon on hand to scoop a tablespoon out when you need it. Use on hands that don't have rings on them because the lotion is thick.

Cardamom and Vanilla Moisturizing Bath Soak

The most important thing to do, if your skin is dry, is to make sure you moisturize after you get out of the tub or shower. In fact, you should dry yourself off as little as possible. Instead, soak in this moisturizing tub, then, when you get out, pat yourself dry, use a moisturizer, and then get dressed.

LEVEL: Easy
MAKES: 1 bath

Ingredients

¼ cup sweet almond oil

10 drops cardamom essential oil

10 drops vanilla essential oil

As the water is running, and the tub is almost filled, pour the ingredients under the running water.

Blue Tansy Bath Bomb

Blue Tansy will help skin that has been made red by inflammation. Native to Morocco, it is rare and part of the chamomile family. It is bright yellow and will add some color to your bath water.

LEVEL: Easy

MAKES: 4 Easter-egg sized molds

Ingredients

8 ounces baking soda

4 ounces Epsom salt

4 ounces corn starch

4 ounces citric acid

2 to 3 tablespoons castor oil

1 tablespoon water

15 drops blue tansy essential oil

10 drops helichrysum essential oil

natural food coloring (optional)

1. In a large bowl, whisk together the baking soda, Epsom salt, corn starch, and citric acid. Keep a silicone mold with 12 forms nearby.

2. In a separate bowl, mix the castor oil, water, essential oils, and, food coloring, if using. Use only a single color of food coloring to guarantee that the bath water won't turn brown.

3. Very slowly, add the liquid to the dry mixture, whisking as you do so. The result should be a mixture that feels like damp sand.

4. Immediately put the mixture into the silicone molds. Press the mixture firmly into the molds before it begins to dry.

5. Cover the mold if you're using one that isn't ball/sphere-shaped and let the mixture dry for 24 hours.

Warming Hand Sugar Scrub

This is a wonderful winter scrub for dry hands. To make a matching hand cream for this scrub, use the recipe for the Moisturizing Red Apple and Rose Intensive Hand Cream on page 128 and swap out those two essential oils for the three in this recipe.

LEVEL: Easy

MAKES: 1 use

Ingredients

2 tablespoons brown sugar

1 tablespoon olive oil

5 drops vanilla essential oil

2 drops ginger essential oil

2 drops cinnamon essential oil

Mix all ingredients in a bowl. Rub on your hands and "wash" with the scrub. Be gentle and rinse well.

Family

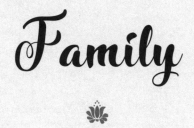

Cedarwood Rollerball Deodorant

In the hot yoga classes I attend, there are frequently men in my classes and they sure do sweat. A lot. Sweating is good for you, but it is very difficult to ignore the aroma of sweating men. I created this deodorant to make the room smell a little more pleasant for everyone, so its scent is subtle because the truth is, you can't mask body odor with a very strong scent. If you try to, you only get two strong scents. It's better to try to have them mingle together gently.

LEVEL: Easy

MAKES: 1 (10-milliliter) roller bottle

Ingredients

10 drops cedarwood essential oil

2 tablespoons grapeseed oil

1. Combine all ingredients in the bowl. Stir gently.

2. Funnel the liquid into a glass roller bottle.

3. Use as you would other deodorant.

Valerian Root Herbal Pet Shampoo

I am a dog lover, and all of my dogs have loved to be outside with me. I also live in a state with a lot of ticks, so before we come back inside, I give my dogs a quick rinse and check for ticks, which is easier to do when their fur is wet. I have small dogs, so if you have big dogs, you'll have to double (or triple!) the recipes. Also, I use a hose, so I haven't included water in the recipe. This shampoo has valerian root, which has relaxation effects, so if your dog might be less reactive if he typically doesn't like getting baths or gets nervous if you find a tick and have to remove it.

LEVEL: Easy

MAKES: 1 (18-ounce) glass bottle

Ingredients

2 cups apple cider vinegar

½ cup liquid Castile soap

20 drops valerian root essential oil

10 drops lemongrass essential oil

1. Mix all ingredients in a liquid measuring cup.

2. Use a hose or showerhead to spray your dog so that he's wet.

3. Pour some shampoo on the dog's back and lather. Check for ticks by running your hands all over his body, especially in crevices. Turn the hose on gently and use the water to move the fur or hair around so you can see the skin. Remove any ticks.

4. Rinse all the shampoo from your dog.

Ylang-Ylang Date Night Shampoo

In my experience, whether you're going out on a first date, a third date, or the thousandth date, your scent is enticing only if it is subtle. Although I adore fragrance (obviously), I try not to overdo it when I'm going to be close to someone, and I've found that nicely scented shampoo and soap are ideal. Like most projects in this book, you can give this as a gift, or use it as make-and-take project, letting everyone decide what oils they want to use as their personal fragrance. Don't forget to put personalized labels on the bottles.

LEVEL: Easy

MAKES: 1 (16-ounce) glass bottle

Ingredients

- 1 cup liquid Castile soap
- ¼ cup aloe vera juice
- ¼ cup apple cider vinegar
- 20 drops ylang-ylang essential oil

1. Add all the ingredients into a shampoo bottle. Shake gently until mixed.

2. Apply to hair and shampoo as you normally would. You will have to shake each time you use, as the ingredients may separate.

Cooling Bubble Bath for Kids

Kids love summer and summer makes them extra dirty, which is part of the fun for them! Frequently, when we think of bubble baths, we assume the water will be warm, but this bubble bath features oils that are cooling. Of course, your children won't want to get into a cold bath, but the water can be just below hot and the oils will give the sensation of cooling.

LEVEL: Easy

MAKES: 1 bath

Ingredients

- ½ cup Castile soap
- 10 drops spearmint essential oil
- 10 drops lemongrass essential oil

When the tub is almost filled, pour the soap into the tub, and then add the oils.

Anti-Insect Pet Spray

I am always hesitant to have my dog wear anti-tick collars or to spray him with the chemicals that fight ticks, especially because my dog sleeps with me and I don't want the chemicals that close to me. Nevertheless, I need to keep the ticks off my dog, because where we live, there are a lot of tick-borne diseases. This spray has been a lifesaver (but note that no treatment is guaranteed to prevent ticks or other insect bites). I spray it on my dog before we go outside. I created this recipe for a 20-pound dog, so use less if your pet is smaller. Just like with babies and children, always err on the side of caution and use less at first. You can always add more if you feel you need a higher concentration. Many tick repellent recipes call for citronella essential oil, but I do not use that because it is highly toxic for cats, and that makes me think it might not be healthy for any animal.

LEVEL: Easy

MAKES: 1 (4-ounce) spray bottle

Ingredients

4 tablespoons sweet almond oil

4 tablespoons apple cider vinegar

5 drops orange essential oil

5 drops geranium essential oil

5 drops lavender essential oil

1. Put all the ingredients into the glass bottle. Shake gently.

2. Spray on your animal before he goes outside.

3. When your pet comes inside, rinse him off or, at the very least, wipe him down with a washcloth and check him for ticks.

Orange and Lemongrass School Focus Candle

This would be a great project to do with a Scout troop, either girls or boys. This is also a great activity for an environmental badge because this recipe uses old candles and old milk cartons.

LEVEL: Hard

MAKES: 1 candle

Ingredients

used unscented candles, crushed

double boiler

large ice cubes

1 wick

Pencils

empty and rinsed milk carton

5 drops sweet orange essential oil

5 drops lemongrass essential oil

1. Put the old candles in a double boiler to melt the wax.

2. Cut the wick so that it is long enough to hang all the way down the milk carton while a good bit of each is wrapped and tied around a pencil. Put the pencil with the wick across the top of the milk carton.

3. Put ice cubes in the milk carton.

4. Pour the melted wax over the ice and let the wax harden while the ice melts. This will take just a few minutes.

5. Pour the water from the ice out of the carton and peel the carton away from the candle.

6. Unwrap the wick from the pencil and cut the wick if it's too long for the candle.

7. Light the wick, and study!

Eucalyptus and Camphor Rollerball Chest Congestion Soother

Eucalyptus and Camphor are wonderful to open the chest and breathing passages. Using a small rollerball is an easy way to put this under your child's nose, and it doesn't have petroleum like the over-the-counter decongestant products. To use, roll the oil just under the nose and on the chest. Put a T-shirt on a baby or child so they don't get it on their hands.

LEVEL: Easy

MAKES: 1 (10 milliliter) roller bottle

Ingredients

40 drops eucalyptus essential oil

25 drops camphor essential oil

40 drops wintergreen essential oil

teaspoon jojoba oil

Add all ingredients to the roller bottle, close the bottle, and shake gently to combine.

Baby Bottom Soother

Even the best cared-for babies sometimes get diaper rash, especially if they have been playing in sand or sitting in a stroller for a long time. It's awful to see your baby's bottom red and sore. I want to remind you that you should never use an undiluted essential oil on the broken skin of a baby. Your goal is to use a soothing cream. Many diaper rash creams have zinc oxide, which soothes broken skin, and homemade ones can only use this ingredient. You can buy pure zinc oxide cream at the drugstore or health food store and then add a very small drop of essential oils to the cream.

LEVEL: Medium

MAKES: 1 small Mason jar

Ingredients

4 teaspoons zinc oxide cream

2 teaspoons beeswax

2 drops lavender essential oil

2 drops tea tree essential oil

1. Mix all the ingredients in a bowl. Transfer mixture to a glass jar, and cover tightly.

2. As needed, put a very small amount on your baby's bottom. You only need a thin layer.

Soothe the Gums Teething Oil

Tooth pain is excruciating, both for adults and for babies. Don't hesitate to let your baby chew on teething toy, because the pressure actually takes away the pain sensation. Teething crackers are also good, too. Like you would do with any product that your baby might ingest, be sure you are using food-grade oils.

LEVEL: Easy

MAKES: 1 small dropper bottle

Ingredients

3 tablespoons olive oil

10 drops chamomile essential oil

1. Wash your hands with unscented hand soap.

2. Put the olive oil and the essential oil into a dropper bottle. Shake gently.

3. Drop a bit on your finger and run your finger gently along your child's gums.

TIP: If your child seems to like the taste of chamomile, make a cup of chamomile tea and soak a clean washcloth in the tea. When it's cool (or even cold; you can put it in the refrigerator) let your baby chew or suck on it. Chamomile is calming.

Baby Shampoo and Soap

I never wanted to be a preachy mother (and, for the most part, I'm not), but using store-bought shampoos is little better than putting laundry detergent on your child. Of course, there are good alternatives, like this recipe. If your child's hair tangles frequently, use the Geranium Hair Detangler Spray on page 109 to separate the strands and comb more easily.

LEVEL: Easy

MAKES: 1 (24-ounce) bottle

Ingredients

1½ cups unscented Castile soap

2 tablespoons fractionated coconut oil

2 teaspoons water

15 drops lavender essential oil

15 drops chamomile essential oil

5 drops peppermint essential oil

1. Add all ingredients to a plastic shampoo bottle. Shake gently.

2. To use, put a dime-sized amount in your hand, rub your hands together, and spread throughout your baby's hair. Use your fingertips to rub their scalp gently. Cover the baby's eyes when you rinse.

TIP: Normally I put all essential oil make-and-takes in glass bottles, but it is safer to use plastic near babies, especially in the tub where things can easily slip and break.

Calming Rollerball

The most important thing to know about using essential oils with babies is that you need very little. Also, make sure to apply it somewhere that they can't touch, such as their backs. Remember that our skin absorbs the oil, so you want to use oils that are considered food safe (although, that doesn't mean you should feed an oil to a baby; I certainly wouldn't).

LEVEL: Easy

MAKES: 1 small roller bottle

Ingredients

15 drops lavender essential oil

5 drops cedarwood essential oil

5 drops chamomile essential oil

1 teaspoon sweet almond oil

1. Put all the ingredients in a small roller bottle and close tightly.

2. Use rollerball on the baby's back or on another area they are unlikely to touch, such as the back of the upper arms, neck, top of the head, or back of the legs. You can also put the scent on a cloth that rests on the crib, out of reach.

Cat Deterrent Spray

Cats are notoriously repelled by citrus scents, so you can use virtually any citrus essential oil in this mix to put where your cats tend to scratch. Be sure to first test this recipe on hidden parts of your couch to be sure it doesn't stain the fabric, and you might even consider using it solely on parts of your couch that aren't visible, such as under the cushions or even under the couch. The scent will still be obvious to your pets.

LEVEL: Easy

MAKES: 1 (8-ounce) spray bottle

Ingredients

¼ cup water

¼ cup witch hazel

20 drops lemon essential oil

10 drops eucalyptus essential oil

1. Pour all ingredients a spray bottle and shake gently to mix.

2. Spray on non-visible parts of couch or furniture where your cat tends to scratch.

TIP: Scratching is good for cats so you don't want to stop them from doing it all together. To train them to scratch better locations, such as a box or scratching post, put sachets of catnip on the areas you want them to scratch, as your cat will probably choose the scent of catnip over the scent of the couch with the spray.

Cedarwood Anti-Anxiety Pet Spray

My son and I once had a beagle named Rocket (so named because he took off from us like a rocket when we brought him to the beach) and when we weren't home, he barked and barked. Some dogs, like our current one, Morty, like to be home, but others, like Rocket, become very anxious when left by themselves. This spray was recommended to me by our vet.

LEVEL: Easy

MAKES: 1 (4-ounce) spray bottle

Ingredients

3 tablespoons distilled water

3 tablespoons witch hazel

20 drops cedarwood essential oil

20 drops frankincense essential oil

Small spray bottle

1. Pour all ingredients into a small spray bottle. Shake gently to combine.

2. Spray a bit on your dog's bed and on the places where they commonly sleep.

Sandalwood and Lavender Shave Cream

Perhaps this is a little sexist, but most of the recipes I labeled "men" have a woodsy scent, but there are many floral scents that pair well with woodsy oils, such as violet and lavender, which is the one I chose for those shave cream. It works perfectly well on legs, too.

LEVEL: Medium

MAKES: 1 (4-ounce) bottle

Ingredients

1 tablespoon avocado oil

1 cup avocado oil

3 tablespoons Castile soap

1 teaspoon vitamin E oil

10 drops of sandalwood essential oil

15 drops of lavender essential oil

bowl

hand mixer

Mason jar

1. Put your bowl in the freezer for a few minutes, then take it out. Using your hand mixer, combine all the ingredients in the cold bowl for two to three minutes. The mixture should be light and fluffy.

2. Put the cream in the Mason jar.

3. Your cream may melt a little if you keep it in your bathroom. You can re-whip or keep it in the fridge.

Men's Eucalyptus Deodorant

Eucalyptus is very aromatic, but it is an herbal scent, so it is a great scent for men to use, especially if they don't like woody scents.

LEVEL: Medium

MAKES: 1 tube

Ingredients

¼ cup baking soda

¼ cup corn starch

2 tablespoons shea butter

15 drops eucalyptus essential oil

15 drops tea tree essential oil

Combine all ingredients in a medium bowl. Once well combined, press the mixture firmly into the empty deodorant tube and let rest in refrigerator for an hour so it solidifies more firmly. Use as you would any other antiperspirant.

White Fir Beard Oil

With the artisan/crafts movement coming along at the same time as the beard revival movement, using essential oils to make mixtures for men is actually a possibility. When I first started experimenting with beard recipes, I went online and was amused to find that rather than using liquid measuring cups, the male writers of the recipes used one ounce shot glasses. Clever, no?

LEVEL: Easy

MAKES: 1 (1-ounce) dropper bottle

Ingredients

1 teaspoon jojoba oil

1 teaspoon sweet almond oil

5 drops white fir essential oil

5 drops tea tree essential oil

1. Put the oils in a dropper bottle, cover, and shake gently to mix.

2. To use, put a couple of drops on your fingers after a shower and thoroughly rub into your beard.

White Fir Beard Softener

This cream is made for men with sturdier beards, and who would like their hair to be soft, not scratchy, stiff, or slick. This recipe requires a little more work than the beard oil, but it may be the perfect gift for the gentleman in your life.

LEVEL: Medium

MAKES: 1 (2-ounce) bottle

Ingredients

4 tablespoons fractionated coconut oil

1 tablespoon sweet almond oil

20 drops white fir essential oil

10 drops peppermint essential oil

1. Put the coconut oil and Sweet Almond oil in the top of the double boiler, over a low heat, until it melts.

2. Take the sweet almond oil mixture off the heat, put it in a medium bowl, and put the bowl in the refrigerator for a half hour to chill.

3. Take the bowl out of the fridge, add the essential oils, and use a hand blender to make the balm light and frothy. Put the balm in a Mason jar.

4. To use, take a little of the balm and spread on your hands, and then spread throughout your beard.

TIP: If you use the balm or other beard oil every day, your beard may eventually need to be shampooed. Using one of the shampoos made with essential oils will be easier on your facial skin than most commercial shampoos, many of which contain detergents.

Cedarwood Aftershave

I wrote this as a men's recipe, but the truth is, you can swap in any essential oil for the scent so that it will appeal to all genders and gender-fluid people. Scent is personal, and while every essential oil has its specific health benefits, we choose many of them based on scent. Therefore, because almost all adults shave, this recipe will work for anyone and you can use the essential oil combination of your choice to make it uniquely your own. I also enjoy using white apple and rose, white fir and wintergreen, or sweet orange and clove for this recipe. I also always add chamomile, as it's a wonderful skin soother. Leave out the witch hazel if you want less of a tingly feeling.

LEVEL: Easy

MAKES: 1 (4-ounce) bottle

Ingredients

3 tablespoons witch hazel

3 tablespoons aloe vera lotion

3 tablespoons jojoba oil

10 drops cedarwood essential oil

5 drops patchouli essential oil

5 drops chamomile essential oil

Put all ingredients in a Mason jar. Gently shake to combine. To use, pour out a quarter-sized bit in your palm and rub on the area you shaved.

Paw Cream for Doggies

Winter can be tough a dog's paws, as many people put down salt that can burn their paws. When you come in from a walk, use a washcloth to wipe your dog's paws and then put this cream on his feet. Make sure all the essential oils you buy for this recipe are food-grade, although for safety's sake, I put this cream on my dog's feet, let it soak in while I sit with him, and then wipe off as much excess as I can because I don't want him to lick and ingest too much of these (or any non-food) ingredients. (Of course, my dog, like many dogs, will eat many disgusting things, so something like this is probably relatively healthy for my little scavenger!)

LEVEL: Hard

MAKES: 1 small Mason jar

Ingredients

4 tablespoons cocoa butter

1 tablespoon aloe vera gel

1 tablespoon melted beeswax

1 tablespoon olive oil

10 drops rosemary oil

5 drops lavender oil

1. Put the cocoa butter, aloe vera, beeswax, and olive oil in the top of a double boiler over low heat. Once the mixture melts and combines, take it off the stove.

2. Add the essential oils to the cocoa butter mixture, stir to combine, and then put the mixture into a Mason jar. Place the cream in the refrigerator so it will solidify.

Essential
Oil FAQ

What are essential oils?

Essential oils are the aromatic compounds within plants, including the bark, stems, leaves, seed, roots, and flowers. They are called essential because the oils are the "essence" of the plant. A rose wouldn't be a rose without its distinctive scent, or essence, in the same way basil or a lemon always smells like basil and lemon. There are about 200 essential oils, although some are rarer than others, meaning they are expensive and hard to use in our everyday lives.

Essential oils are also volatile, which means they quickly evaporate, and that's why, when you open a bottle, the scent immediately fills the room. It is also why you can use just a few drops of any essential oil in a diffuser or candle, or even just a culinary application, and the scent will linger in the air for a while.

How are essential oils different from other oils, like olive and canola?

Essential oils, unlike food oils, are not the actually oils from a plant. Volatile essential oils are the compounds that remain after certain plant parts are distilled. However, essential oils aren't truly oils; they are only called that because, like oil, the compounds do not mix easily with water

Food oils aren't as aromatic as essential oils. You can open a large bottle of olive oil, for example, and detect the scent of olives, but if you had that large of a bottle of rose oil or ginger oil, the scent would be overwhelming and, in truth, unpleasant.

Does it matter who makes my essential oil?

Yes. As with any product, not all producers sell the same quality essential oil. There aren't strict Food and Drug Administration (FDA) regulations for essential oils, so you might see the words "pure" or "certified" and think that means they are the best you can buy. You can go online and research the quality of the brand name and quality of the oils you want to buy, and you can also get information from the seller, if you buy oils from someone's home.

What is a carrier oil?

Because essential oils are so volatile, and you only need a small amount at a time, they are most often placed in a carrier oil, which is a fragrance-free oil that "carries" the essential oil and its scent. Carrier oils both dilute essential oils (without changing their benefits) and stop them from evaporating too quickly.

Carrier oils do not have the same therapeutic benefits as essential oils. However, they can have other therapeutic values. For example, almond oil is wonderfully moisturizing. Not all vegetarian oils are good as carriers. Mineral oil, for example, is "natural," but it's not good for your skin (despite what it may say on the bottle). Not all carrier oils are actual oils. Some are lotions or creams, and even the oils themselves vary widely in the way they feel and work. Just like you can experiment with essential oils, you also need to experiment with your carriers!

Most essential oil companies sell their own proprietary carrier oils, which are combinations of a number oils, such as wheat germ, coconut, and almond.

Common carrier oils include:

- ❧ Apricot Kernel Oil: A light, sweet oil that does not leave any greasy residue behind and has a lot of oleic and linoleic acid, making it a good anti-inflammatory.

- ❧ Avocado Oil: With its high viscosity, avocado oil is best blended with another carrier. It has high concentrations of oleic and linoleic fatty acids, and vitamins A, D, and E. Avocado can help with psoriasis and eczema.

- ❧ Castor Oil: Castor oil is being rediscovered as more is being learned about its ability to fight bacteria and germs. It contains ricinoleic acid and can be ingested (and has wonderful medicinal value on its own).

🌿 Cocoa Butter: Solid and difficult to work with at room temperature, cocoa butter is best used when melted and blended with other carrier oils. It has a sweet, chocolate aroma.

🌿 Coconut Oil: Solid and white at room temperature with a distinct coconut aroma, coconut oil leaves an oily feeling layer on top of the skin. It has a long shelf life. Fractionated coconut oil is liquid at room temperature and has no noticeable aroma. It absorbs well and feels more silky than oily on the skin. It is high in essential fatty acids and has a long shelf life.

🌿 Grapeseed Oil: Light and with a thin consistency, grapeseed oils is good for massages, but has a short shelf life. It leaves a light film on the skin and is moisturizing. High in linoleic acid, which is a healthy fatty acid.

🌿 Sweet Almond: Slightly sweet with a nutty aroma and a medium consistency, the skin absorbs sweet almond oil quickly. It is rich in vitamin E and oleic acid. It is an excellent all-purpose carrier oil, but it may cause a reaction in people who have a nut allergy.

🌿 Jojoba Oil: With a slight nut aroma and a medium consistency, jojoba oil is also one of the best all-purpose carrier oils because it has a long shelf life. It is non-greasy on the skin because it is similar to the skin's natural oils, and it can moisturize skin and hair.

🌿 Olive Oil: Popular, easy-to-find oil used which can be used on the body or in recipes that are ingested. It is thicker than most oils and rests heavily on the skin, so isn't a great choice for massages. It can also have a strong aroma. Olive oil is healthy and a good source of oleic acid, which is a fatty acid. Like many food oils, it has a relatively short shelf life.

🌿 Shea Butter: Like cocoa butter, shea butter is solid at room temperature and is cream colored. It has a nutty aroma, and is an excellent and effective moisturizer for skin and hair. However, it leaves a waxy-feeling on the skin.

How are essential oils made?

There are two common ways to make essential oils: Distillation and Expression (cold press).

Most oils that you will buy come from companies that use steam to distill their oils. The herbs or flowers are put in boiling water and the oil separates from the water. In this process, steam heated between 140°F and 212°F, depending on the plant, passes through the plant material and the combination of heat and pressure causes microscopic sacs within the plant to release the essential oil. Next, the vapor and the oil flow through a condenser and cool, which causes the essential oil to separate from the water, which is called hydrosol or floral water. The essential oil and the hydrosol are both collected by the manufacturer.

Most essential oils distillation production stops there, but some of the most valuable oils, such as rose or ylang-ylang, are sometimes distilled slightly differently, so you might see the word "absolute." This type of distillation requires higher temperatures and pressure.

Other companies use a cold press method, in which the plants are pressed to get the oil out. Have you ever squeezed an orange rind and felt the oil come out and been able to smell the intense scent? That is expression. This method mechanically presses fruits in order to get their essential oils out. It works well with fruit rinds.

Technically, you can distill and express oils on your own if you want. The machinery isn't that expensive, although growing enough flowers and plants is complicated.

How do I use an essential oil diffuser, and what kind should I buy?

Essential oil diffusers are the easiest and least expensive ways to use essential oils. There are four different types of essential oil diffusers:

✿ Heat: These types of diffusers use various types of heating elements to cause the essential oil to slowly evaporate. It's sort of like spraying an essential oil on a lamp or light bulb to diffuse the scent in a room. This is not the best or most efficient way to use essential oils, though, even though it is often inexpensive. Depending on the source of heat, the scent of the essential oil can change and that is a sign that the therapeutic benefit of the oil may change.

- ❦ Nebulizer: Using an air stream and nozzle, nebulizing diffusers break down an essential oil into tiny particles, which are released into the air as fine mist. This process doesn't change the essential oils at all. Nebulizers are very effective, but they are expensive to buy and to run, as they use more essential oils than the other diffusers.

- ❦ Ultrasonic: One of the most common diffusers available, ultrasonic diffusers use water and a small vibrating disk to create a fine mist of essential oils. This means you can use less of each essential oil, but you get a weaker scent. The machine also acts as a humidifier in the room.

- ❦ Vapor: Using a fan blowing through a filter, this diffuser uses air to help the oil evaporate. This isn't the most effective way to diffuse essential oils because the air dries the oil and the oil rarely evaporates evenly, so you get bursts of different scents depending on the oil or the mixture.

Be sure to follow the directions of whatever type of diffuser you use. The oils will eventually build up and keep it from working properly, so you'll need to make sure you take good care of your equipment. Always clean your diffusers before you switch oils. Sometimes the diffusers will need careful cleaning with a cotton swab and rubbing alcohol. No matter the diffuser, remember that you will need to test every oil to get the scent intensity you want. Working with essential oils is always part experiment.

Are essential oils poisonous?

No oils sold through reputable companies are poisonous, but all essential oils are very concentrated and meant to be used in small amounts in recipes that cut down their power. For example, it takes hundreds of peppermint leaves to make a small bit of the essential oil, and one drop of peppermint essential oil is the equivalent of many cups of the same tea, made also from the leaves. Like anything, too much of a good thing can be unhealthy. Most essential oils should be diluted and not used directly on the skin straight from the bottle. The safest way to use them is aromatically.

For example, I'm a yoga teacher, and frequently I will put some essential oil in my hands, rub my hands together, and then, while my students are in savasana, I might move my hands over their face or gently press on their shoulders to further relax them, but I never put a large amount of the oil on someone's skin. In fact, I may decide not to touch someone directly on their skin if there is oil on my hands, and I always wash my hands after I use essential oils.

The general rule is that an essential oil should be diluted in a carrier oil like jojoba or almond oil in a ratio of 3–5 drops of essential oils per teaspoon of carrier oil, and much less if using on a baby or child. Safety and dilution are linked, just like the strength of alcoholic drink. A lower dilution is generally safer. Also, diluting essential oils is economical; oils are typically expensive. Typically, for a dilution of 1%, add 1 drop of oil to 5 ml of a carrier oil. Multiply this dilution as needed for your recipes.

What oils react to the skin?

Some people are allergic to essential oils, and they won't know it until they have the reaction. So, it is important to be particularly careful with certain essential oils. Citrus oils are known to cause photosensitivity, which means that if you put them on your skin and go out in the sun, you might get burned. Though the risk of photosensitivity varies based on the way the oil was distilled, it is best to not use them on the skin. Citrus oils include orange, lime, lemon, bergamot, and grapefruit. Other oils to look out for are clove bud, and basil: clove bud oil should never be used at a distillation of more than 0.5%, and basil oil at no more than 1%.

If you're going to sell or promote essential oils at a make-and-take party, test each sample one on your skin, such as on your arm, just to get a sense of its strength and how you react to the oil. Or, always have fragrance test strips for your customers to use.

Are essential oils edible?

Some essential oils are edible, but you should assume that whatever you're buying isn't edible, and then do further research to see if it is. I have to say, while I have made products using edible essential oils, I would never offer them to guests at a party, nor would I have them make those products at my party. If I am responsible for people when they are at my house, I want to be safe not sorry. Also, I want to model good habits around essential oils around my guests.

While many essential oils are considered GRAS, or Generally Recognized as Safe, for food and cosmetic use, they have not been studied, especially in concentrated internal amounts, for internal consumption. Many other food ingredients, like salt and sugar, are also considered GRAS, but you wouldn't eat a rollerball full of them!

In many cases, the same benefits of an essential oil can be obtained by using the herb itself, either fresh or dried. For example, I drink a lot of peppermint tea when my seasonal indoor allergies hit because the minty aroma with the combination of hot water is just as, if not more, soothing to me as inhaling the essential oil. During the same time of year, I also drink a lot of hot water with lemon and maple syrup. There is no reason to use an essential oil in place of the actual lemon.

Should essential oils be used as antibiotics?

Remember that essential oils are extremely potent plant compounds that many people think have antibacterial, antimicrobial, antiviral, and antifungal properties. While these are positive qualities—it's great to use tea tree oil to clean your yoga mat—you need to remember that you wouldn't clean your face with the same product you use to clean your yoga mat.

Here's why: Unlike your yoga mat, your body is not dirty. It has bacteria and microbes that are good, and you don't want to affect the bacteria that are keeping you healthy. Because so much of this science is new, very few studies have been conducted about the effects of essential oils on helpful bacteria or on the antibacterial properties of essential oils compared to antibiotics.

On the other hand, antibiotics can be life-saving and it would be absolutely wrong to advice a customer to use an essential oil instead of a medicine that has been prescribed to them. So, if essential oils can behave like antibiotics, we need to exercise the same caution in using them internally.

Are some people allergic to essential oils?

Since essential oils are parts of plants and foods, they can be allergens for people, just like the plants and foods. If you're having a party or using essential oils in public, such as a yoga class, tell everyone in the room before you use them. Ask if anyone is allergic. Be cautious and think the way teachers have to these days: don't use almond oil on people you don't know, for example. There are plenty of safer options.

How do essential oils can change my mood?

It's not the essential oil that changes your mood, but the scent. The emotional reactors in our brains respond to aromas in the same way they respond to a smiling baby or a playful puppy. Scent makes us happy (or nervous, such as in the case of the smell of a skunk). When we smell a pleasant scent or a scent that reminds us of something (such as Doublemint gum, which always reminds me of my mother) our bodies release endorphins (helping us to relax) and serotonin (a mood-booster). Just like our other senses, scent is directly related to our brains and thus our mood.

How long have essential oils been around?

Essential oils have been around for as long as we have known about plants and fruits and herbs, but they probably weren't quite like the ones we use today. Although it was always possible to squeeze a lemon and get the oil out of the rind, it would have been difficult to extract neroli from the orange flower in quite the way we do so now, although most historians think it became available in the 17th century.

The history of perfume is closely entwined with the history of essential oils, and perfumes date back to ancient Egypt, where the use of oils was part of ritual. The scent would have been much lighter back then because modern technology allows manufacturers to get more of the oil than the human-powered methods of the past.

How should I care for my bottles of essential oils?

Essential oils should always be stored in glass vials or bottles. Essential oils are "living" and they don't react well to plastics. Some of them will eat through the plastic, or at least cause it to begin to dissolve, and the plastic can cause the oil to change scent.

If I'm just starting out, which essential oils should I buy first?

We all respond to essential oils in different ways—scent is highly personal, so you need to smell a lot of essential oils to see which ones you like. I adore the scent of rose, while my mother dislikes it, and while I will stand over my lily-of-the-valleys in the spring just sniffing them, I try not to buy perfume with that scent, because it's a little too sweet and youthful for me.

When picking out essential oils, especially if you are considering combining them on your own, you need to consider which ones have longer-lasting aromas. Keep in mind that this will be the main scent.

Next, some oils are complements or "harmonizers." That is, they work well with the primary oils. Sometimes these are oils, like lavender, that are beneficial in many ways and play well with others; in other words, a little bit can hang in the background of another scent. Lavender is strong. so you may smell it even if you use a little behind more drops of a stronger scent, such as rose.

Can I use oils safely when I'm pregnant?

Yes and no. It is perfectly safe to use almost all oils as aromatherapy when pregnant, but I would never advise anyone to take an essential oil internally while pregnant or nursing. Essential oils can affect hormones and stomach bacteria, so it's not wise to use them while you're pregnant and nursing.

Almost all pregnant women use lotions and creams when they are pregnant (so good to keep the skin moisturized) and many of those lotions and creams feature essential oils in them, however, many of those pre-made lotions and creams have gone through rigorous testing, and the essential oils are diluted.

You can, of course, use the recipes in this book to make your own lotions, but you should be completely sure of the safety of your essential oil (and carrier) and know which oils are not safe for pregnant women to use topically. These include fennel, clary sage, marjoram, tarragon, caraway, cinnamon, birch, wintergreen, basil, camphor, hyssop, aniseed, sage, tansy, wormwood, parsley seed or leaf, and pennyroyal.

Having said that, it is perfectly safe for a pregnant woman to inhale peppermint or ginger to see if relieves symptoms of nausea. Likewise, if a pregnant is having trouble sleeping, using lavender in a diffuser or in an eye pillow is in no way harmful.

How do I make sure oils are safe for kids?

Sometimes I see essential oils being touted as "miracle cures" for temper tantrums and crying, and it makes me nervous because nothing is a miracle cure and, like anything, essential oils need to be used judiciously, especially when it comes to children.

Essential oils should never be given as food to children or used undiluted on their skin. They should be diluted more than they are for adults, and they should never be put directly on children or baby's skin.

Typically, lavender, chamomile, orange, and lemon are considered safe for diluted use on children, but I would always do a skin test first. Surprisingly, some seemingly common oils, such as peppermint, rosemary, eucalyptus, and wintergreen are considered unsafe for babies and young children. Most importantly, because a child is young, you don't yet know what each child may be allergic to.

Can I make my own sunscreen with essential oil?

There are a lot of recipes available online and in other books for all-natural sunscreens made with zinc oxide, but I didn't feel comfortable publishing a recipe for one because I can't guarantee its effectiveness. Zinc oxide is definitely an effective physical barrier against the sun's rays, but when a product is homemade, you can't definitely know its sun protection factor (SPF) or effectiveness.

I have offered a few recipes with zinc in them, specifically diaper rash cream, which has long been a skin soother for babies, but, of course, in that area, it isn't being used for sun protection. Because zinc oxide is not water soluble, it is good agent at blocking out water (and urine) to help a baby's skin heal.

Can I use essential oils in gardening?

I only made a few recipes for the garden, but, essential oils have been shown to be very effective in gardens. Oils including clove, lavender, and tea tree are insect repellents, and some, such as pine, repel fleas and ticks. Rosemary keeps flies and mosquitoes away, and peppermint repels almost everything, including spiders.

If you are a gardener, my suggestion would be to get a library of essential oils and start your own experiments, spraying them around a variety of plants to see which ones are most effective with your garden, soil, bugs, and insects.

Acknowledgments

It is always an honor to work with a wonderful team of editors and designers, but it is especially wonderful when everyone is nice and helpful and supportive, and that has been the case with Ulysses. Thank you, Casie Vogel, for your enthusiasm and positive attitude. Shayna Keyles shaped this book and I appreciate her insight and hard work. Claire Sielaff moved the book along swiftly and Claire Chun also raised the quality of the work. Thank you, too, to Raquel Castro for the cover design.

About the Author

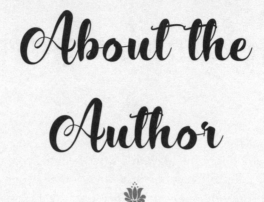

Donna Raskin, a health and fitness writer, is a yoga teacher and adjunct writing professor at The College of New Jersey. The author of *Yoga Beats the Blues* and many other books, she has written for *Shape*, *Cooking Light*, *Men's Health*, and numerous other publications. A lifelong lover of all things fragrant, Ms. Raskin uses essential oils to create cleaning products, sachets, candles, and lotions. She is most drawn to the aromas of lily of the valley, rose, bergamot, and eucalyptus.